Applied Drama and Theatre as an Interdisciplinary Field in the Context of HIV/AIDS in Africa

Matatu
Journal for African Culture and Society

- *Matatu* is a journal on African and African diaspora literatures, cultures, and societies dedicated to interdisciplinary dialogue between literary and cultural studies, historiography, the social sciences, and cultural anthropology.
- *Matatu* is animated by a lively interest in African culture and literature (including the Afro-Caribbean) that moves beyond worn-out clichés of 'cultural authenticity' and 'national liberation' towards critical exploration of African modernities. The East African public transport vehicle from which *Matatu* takes its name is both a component and a symbol of these modernities: based on 'Western' (these days usually Japanese) technology, it is a vigorously African institution; it is usually regarded with some anxiety by those travelling in it, but is often enough the only means of transport available; it creates temporary communicative communities and provides a transient site for the exchange of news, storytelling, and political debate.
- *Matatu* is firmly committed to supporting democratic change in Africa, to providing a forum for interchanges between African and European critical debates, to overcoming notions of absolute cultural, ethnic or religious alterity, and to promoting transnational discussion on the future of African societies in a wider world.

Applied Drama and Theatre as an Interdisciplinary Field in the Context of HIV/AIDS in Africa

Edited by

Hazel Barnes

Rodopi

Amsterdam - New York, NY 2013

Matatu Number 43

Cover image: Rozanne Myburgh

The paper on which this book is printed meets the requirements of "ISO 9706:1994, Information and documentation - Paper for documents - Requirements for permanence".

ISBN: 978-90-420-3806-6
E-Book ISBN: 978-94-012-1053-9

Printed in The Netherlands

Contents

List of Illustrations ix
Acknowledgements xi
Introduction xiii

SETTING THE SCENE

PATRICK MANGENI 3
Negotiating the Space: Challenges for Applied-Theatre Praxis with Local Non-Governmental/Community-Based Organizations in HIV/AIDS Contexts in Uganda

DAVID KERR 31
HIV Communication: Global Emergencies, Media Templates, and African Communities (A Personal Journey)

INNOVATIONS IN RESEARCH APPROACHES

EMELDA NGUFOR SAMBA 47
Appreciative Inquiry – An Alternative Approach to Applied Theatre

GORDON BILBROUGH 61
After the Curtain – Reframed: Using Action Research to Reflect, Monitor, and Evaluate the Applied-Theatre Experience

REBECCA ANN RUGG 83
Collaboration as Research: Yale University, Siwela Sonke Dance Theatre, Clowns Without Borders South Africa, and People's Educational Theatre Swaziland

NEHEMIAH CHIVANDIKWA 109
Participatory Theatre for Development as Action Research: Methodological, Theoretical and Ethical Challenges, Tensions and Possibilities with Specific Reference to an HIV/AIDS and Disability Project (2007–2010)

INNOVATIONS IN HIV/AIDS AWARENESS EDUCATION

DIANA WILSON AND KAREN SUTER 127
The Lover and Another: A Consideration of the Efficacy of Utilizing a Performance Poetry Competition as Vehicle for HIV/AIDS Education Among Young Adults

SELLOANE MOKUKU 145
Do, Be, Do: Insights from 'Rapid Cognition' in a Theatre-Making Process

JOHANNES VISSER 161
Space and Involvement – Theatre in (a) South African Prison

INNOVATIONS IN RESEARCH PRACTICE/THEORY

ALEXANDRA SUTHERLAND 177
Dramatic Spaces in Patriarchal Contexts: Constructions and Disruptions of Gender in Theatre Interventions About HIV

GALIA BONEH 187
This Is My Story: A Model for Creating Performance Engaging Artists and People Living with HIV/AIDS

KENNEDY CHINYOWA 203
A Poetic of Contradictions? HIV/AIDS Interventions at the Crossroads of Localization and Globalization

JAMIE LACHMAN 219
Project Njabulo: Using Storytelling, Drama, and Play Therapy for Psycho-Social Interventions in Communities Affected by HIV/AIDS in Southern Africa – Pathways to Empathetic Locally Sustainable Care

INNOVATIVE CASE STUDIES

MYER TAUB 235
Dramatic Beading

REMO CHIPATISO 251
Evaluation of Applied Drama and Theatre in HIV/AIDS Interventions: A Case Study of Themba Interactive

TENDAI MTUKWA 269
Theatre as Border-Crossing Among Women Living with HIV: A Case Study of Zandspruit Informal Settlement

Notes on Contributors 281
Onomastic Index 285
Notes for Contributors 293

List of Illustrations

EMELDA NGUFOR SAMBA
Figure 1: The four Ds of Cooperrider and Whitney 54

GORDON BILBROUGH
Figure 1: Learning increase, 2006–2008 79

REBECCA ANN RUGG
Figure 1: Student with project mask 89
Figure 2: First-encounter dance 93
Figure 3: Brandon Wheatley and Stanley Mabuza 95
Figure 4: Storyteller figure played by Musawenkosi Zikalala 96
Figure 5: Musa Zikalala's theatre at nKwalini 97
Figure 6: Rehearsal at nKwalini's hillside theatre 97
Figure 7: Street theatre, Durban 101
Figure 8: Street theatre, Durban 102
Figure 9: Musa Zikalala's theatre at nKwalini 105
Figure 10: Performance at nKwalini theatre 105
Figure 11: Clowning at nKwalini theatre 106

SELLOANE MOKUKU
Figure 1: WSI Play-Generation Process 152

GALIA BONEH
Figure 1: "Se Anka Eye Wo a…" 187
Figure 2: "This Is My Story" 187
Figures 3 and 4: Process–Product Balance 189
Figure 5: From Messaging to Critical Thinking 190
Figure 6: Targeting the Community 190

Figures 7 and 8: Victimhood and Compassion 192
Figure 9: Vitality in Performance 192
Figures 10 and 11: Vitality in Performance 193
Figure 12: From Breaking Barriers to Performance 193
Figure 13: This Is My Story 196

JAMIE LACHMAN
Figure 1: CWBSA participatory action research methodology 223
Figure 2: Cycle of Suffering from HIV/AIDS pandemic 225
Figure 3: Intervention Model 1: Basic Transference to Community Level 229
Figure 4: Intervention Model 2: Complete Transference of Skills to Community Level 230

MYER TAUB
Figure 1: Watching video at the Monkeybiz wellness clinic, Cape Town 236
Figure 2: Rhizome models 239
Figure 3: Playing with bags and beads 243
Figure 4: Exploring maps as mapping 246
Figure 5: Mandisa's fourth map 247

Acknowledgements

THANKS TO ALL THE CONTRIBUTORS who have generously submitted their essays and for their willingness to revise their material, and their patience in tolerating what has been a lengthy process of preparation.

Particular thanks to Warren Nebe and Kennedy Chinyowa, who willingly helped with editorial decisions.

The Drama for Life Programme and Africa Research Conferences are the result of the vision of Warren Nebe and the generous support of all the donors, particularly the German Development Corporation and the Goethe-Institut Südafrika and also the National Research Foundation, the University of the Witwatersrand, the Deutscher Entwicklungsdienst, the Higher Education HIV/AIDS Programme, the World Alliance for Arts Education, and Make Art Stop AIDS.

Introduction

THIS BOOK RESULTS FROM RESEARCH initiated or supported by Drama for Life. The Drama for Life Programme within the Division of Dramatic Arts at the University of Witwatersrand School of Arts is a highly innovative and acclaimed programme which has already, in the short time it has been in operation, made an impact through its use of drama and theatre to investigate the effect of HIV/AIDS on communities. The objective of the programme is as follows:

> To enhance the capacity of young people, theatre practitioners and their communities to take responsibility for the quality of their lives in the context of HIV and AIDS in Africa. We achieve this through participatory and experiential drama and theatre that is appropriate to current social realities but draws on the rich indigenous knowledge of African communities.[1]

Drama for Life aims to offer Honours, Masters, and PhD programmes that build capacity in HIV/AIDS education through applied drama and theatre. It provides an opportunity for experienced practitioners to develop their theoretical understanding and skills and to return these to their communities. It draws students from the whole of Southern Africa and as far north as Uganda and Ghana.[2] It enhances the capacity of communities to take responsibility for the quality of their lives through a responsive integrated approach in arts activism, education, research, and therapies which is appropriate to current social realities. The focus is not only on capacity development in HIV/AIDS education, activism, and therapy but also on peace building, transformation and diversity management, and on human rights, social justice, and environmental sustainability.

---

[1] http://www.dramaforlife.co.za/index.php/about (22nd February 2010)

[2] To date, Drama for Life has alumni and scholars from fourteen African countries – Botswana, Cameroon, Ghana, Kenya, Namibia, Swaziland, Lesotho, Mozambique, Malawi, Tanzania, Zambia, South Africa, Uganda and Zimbabwe.

Drama for Life has established two annual events which enable the programme to interface with community practitioners and with applied drama and theatre academics. The first of these is the Drama for Life Festival, which brings together and showcases the performance work of various communities using applied drama and theatre. The Festival aims at finding effective and innovative theatrical expression for the human implications of the AIDS pandemic and to invigorate practice of HIV-related performance. The intention of the Festival is not one of message-giving but, rather, to explore the many ways in which the pandemic has affected people's lives and see how these can find expression through the arts in order to make a meaningful impact on audiences. This public exposure, and the interchange and networking that result from it, is an important stimulus to research and development work through the arts in Africa. The second event is the Drama for Life African Research Conference in Applied Drama and Theatre, which draws scholars from Africa and elsewhere to exchange insights on the theoretical approaches, innovations, and practices of applied drama and theatre on the African continent. It has a particular focus on developing understanding of the practice in Africa and on how indigenous knowledge and practice can be used to enhance and vivify the processes of applied drama and theatre.

The first African Research Conference was held in 2008 and the main objective was to consider ways and means of formalizing the evaluation, analysis, and writing-up of applied drama and theatre practice as an increasingly rigorous and sophisticated praxis. Three themes were identified as being of particular concern to practitioners and researchers in Africa at this stage of its development, where the paradigm of Practice as Research is still being determined. These themes included: What constitutes 'best-practice' research approaches in applied drama and theatre work? What ethical positions, values, and principles could be most appropriate in guiding practitioners, participants, researchers, and other stakeholders in applied drama and theatre practice? What monitoring and evaluation methods/techniques are best suited to assessing the value and impact of applied drama and theatre projects in African contexts?

This conference resulted in the establishment of a network of African Practitioners of Applied Drama and Theatre, and the articulation of an Ethics Charter and a Charter on the Principles for Monitoring and Evaluation in Applied Drama and Theatre.

Collected here, in this volume, is a representative set of research written to facilitate dialogue across disciplines concerning the role of Drama and

Theatre in HIV/AIDS education, prevention, and rehabilitation. The conversations centre on innovative research paradigms and approaches and their interface with other disciplines in an interdisciplinary context of HIV/AIDS.

Drama for Life is a research-driven programme. The intention behind this collection is to give readers a sense of the range of work and of approaches occurring in Africa. While all the work reflected on here has occurred in Africa, a number of the essays reflect intercontinental partnerships (Rugg, Boneh, and Lachman), and such connections to global practice are an important input both in the field and in theorizing best practice.

Through a detailed examination of the problems of nepotism, corruption, and survival within fieldwork in Uganda, PATRICK MANGENI examines the delicate negotiations necessary for the effective application of applied drama and theatre in this context, highlighting the importance of strategic partnerships and of sustainability in work around HIV/AIDS. Attention is drawn particularly to the difficulties involved in researching and evaluating applied drama and theatre. DAVID KERR engages with the ways in which the media are used in HIV/AIDS education and awareness-building, and contrasts the ethos and methodologies of the 'total communication' of the media with the face-to-face interaction of applied drama and theatre. He draws attention to the ways in which 'new media' such as blogs, chat rooms, and cell phones allow users to africanize the imported concepts behind the media edutainment through their personalized dialogue. He provides useful critique, as well as suggestions, on how use of media can be made more appropriate within an African context.

Academic research approaches have the potential to re-invigorate research and develop practice. Drawing on the stimulating influence of global trends in the field, the challenge is to integrate these within an African cultural perspective. EMELDA NGUFOR SAMBA highlights the value of Appreciative Inquiry as a suitable complementary methodology which focuses on what she considers to be a more empowering and energizing approach to problem-solving. GORDON BILBROUGH provides an in-depth study of the application of Action Research to the work of arepp: Theatre for Life, suggesting the effectiveness of careful, ongoing evaluation in the development and sustainability of the project. REBECCA RUGG reports on a project involving four different institutions, and the negotiations and developments around research practice which have resulted from the collaboration, initiating "an evolving model for artistic and pedagogical collaboration through interdisciplinary, multi-institutional, intercultural practice." NEHEMIAH CHIVANDIKWA examines the use of Theatre for Development research methodology in the field of disability activism, classifying it as a form of action research and identifying what these two methodologies can contribute in this field.

Essays by Wilson, Suter, Mokuku, and Visser investigate a number of different methodologies in HIV/AIDS-awareness education. These give a sense of the variety of approaches possible and stimulate further enquiry into effective ways of increasing sensibility that take into account the intricate human issues involved. DIANA WILSON and KAREN SUTER outline the use of Performance Poetry at the University of KwaZulu–Natal as a popular form which encourages an in-depth approach to understanding complex issues involved in sexual relationships as well as drawing-in crowds of interested supporters. SELLOANE MOKUKU investigates the usefulness of Malcolm Gladwell's theory of 'rapid cognition' as part of the improvisatory process used by the international Winter/Summer Institute in Lesotho, identifying the importance of an enabling environment, time pressure, and skilful facilitation as being crucial to its success. JOHANNES VISSER analyses the demands on methodology made by working in the very specific environment of the Pretoria C-Max prison. Drawing on the expertise of a number of different disciplines involved in the project, Visser identifies the particular conditions to be taken into account, outlines the methodology used, and makes suggestions for its development.

In the section "Innovations in Applied Drama and Theatre Theory/ Practice," ALEXANDRA SUTHERLAND supports the call for a move away from the binary opposites of much critical pedagogy. Quoting Jonathan Jansen, she argues "for a pedagogy of hope, where counter-narratives are shown, so as not to essentialize social positions of oppressor and oppressed." Her essay elucidates this position in relation to her practice in the context of gender perceptions amongst adolescents in relation to HIV/AIDS. GALIA BONEH analyses a project undertaken in Ghana and then in Malawi which has the objective of including people living with AIDS in the creation and presentation of theatre. The methodology is investigated in terms of its impact on both performers and audiences and its flexibility over the two different terrains. KENNEDY CHINYO is disturbed by the contradictions between global and local expectations of applied drama and theatre methodology. He analyses these contradictions in relation to the use of folk media, participation, and syncretism, concluding with an appeal for an honest engagement with these problems in order to move away from the sense of loss of agency which they engender. Clowns without Borders, South Africa, is an organization which is making an impact in terms of psycho-social support for communities suffering from AIDS through play, storytelling, clowning, and mindfulness training. JAMIE LACHMAN provides an overview of their work and structure as well as explanations of changes made in their methodology through critical evaluation of their fieldwork.

This volume concludes with three case studies of the use of applied drama and theatre. In the first of these, MYER TAUB examines processes of mapping as a creative device for playmaking in comparison to earlier experimentation with digital stimuli, while, in the second, REMO CHIPATISO evaluates the methodology of Themba Interactive Theatre through an analysis of the various modes of communication used by the company. TENDAI MTUKWA's essay investigates principles of applied drama in the context of women living with HIV in the Zandspruit Informal Settlement. Her research validates the importance of playfulness, both in energizing those in positions of hopelessness and in enabling the distancing essential to observe one's situation and thus find possibilities for change.

This research provides a stimulus for the ongoing investigation of current practice and an invitation for further development of innovative and experimental approaches. Drama for Life, in its active support for research in applied drama and theatre, provides a public platform for the dissemination of praxis and as such is an important goad to increasing the excellence and effectiveness of applied drama and theatre, as well as opening up possibilities for interdisciplinary collaboration.

HAZEL BARNES

⌘

Setting the Scene

Patrick Mangeni

Negotiating the Space

Challenges for Applied-Theatre Praxis with Local Non-Governmental/ Community-Based Organizations in HIV/AIDS Contexts in Uganda

This essay draws on the Uganda context to consider the nature of the space in which applied theatre is situated as an agent for change and education. How might this space inform the nature of applied-theatre praxis in contexts of HIV/AIDS initiatives? How might applied-theatre research be negotiated as a form to enhance understanding and to address the goals of change? I will, however, focus more on discussing applied-theatre initiatives carried out in partnership with local non-governmental organizations (NGOs) and community-based organizations (CBOs). The latter often overlap in category with the former. I will thus use CBO to refer to both types of organization and to differentiate them from international NGOs, which, for the purpose of this discussion, I will refer to as NGOs. In this discussion, I will seek to highlight the nature of the space in which these initiatives are located and the implications of this context on HIV/AIDS initiatives. I have chosen to focus on the CBOs, which, unlike their counterparts, the international NGOs, are characterized by peculiarities that raise a series of questions that we need to reflect on in order to address some of the key challenges that have implications for applied-theatre praxis in general and HIV/AIDS interventions through theatre in particular.

I will briefly situate myself in this context as a teacher, practitioner, and researcher. I draw my analyses partly from my experience as a teacher of applied theatre and a trainer and facilitator of community-theatre groups in collaboration with CBOs and government using theatre to advance health education for development agendas, HIV/AIDS being one of these. I have also drawn on project reports and interviews with practitioners engaged in HIV/AIDS initiatives in partnership with CBOs. I draw much from interviews with Baron Oron, who is one of the leading practitioners in applied theatre in the East African region and is one of the pioneer applied-theatre practitioners who have graduate from Makerere University.[1] Oron has for close to two decades facilitated a number of local and international initiatives using theatre to intervene in HIV/AIDS.

My introduction to the practice of theatre-and-HIV/AIDS education as a collaborative engagement was with the School Health Education Project (SHEP) in Uganda in the early to mid-1990s. This was a project under the then Ministry of Education and Sports and which was supported by UNICEF. This initiative, which I discussed elsewhere in more detail,[2] was a collaboration between the Ministries of Education and Sports (MoES), the Ministry of Health (MoH), UNICEF, and theatre artists. The purpose was mainly to intervene to stem HIV infections in schools and to support positive living among the population infected and affected by HIV/AIDS. In this SHEP project I was co-opted as a member of the national board. Part of our responsibility was to participate in determining the nature of the strategy: planning, and administration of the process aimed at promoting social action against AIDS. We have worked with and through schools and communities developing and or reviewing materials for training and managing the processes of training; developing materials for trainers of trainers, who included district inspectors of schools and representatives from interest groups. These in turn trained school choir masters. We then oversaw the latter, training schoolchildren in playmaking and in the development of productions to respond to HIV/AIDS in the country.

The other categories we have worked with have been facilitators involved in applied-theatre initiatives in AIDS education with various CBOs. These have included graduates of the theatre programme at Makerere University,

---

[1] See an earlier interview with Baron Oron: Patrick Mangeni, "Change in two hours: A theatre for development workshop with high-school students in Kampala," *Researching Drama in Education Journal* 3.1 (1998): 93–96.

[2] Patrick Mangeni, "A Theatrical Alternative for Child Survival: The Experience of School Health Drama in Uganda," in *Drama, Culture and Empowerment*, ed. John O'Toole & Kate Donelan (Brisbane: IDEA Publications, 1996): 77–85.

leaders of satellite groups and associations that are members of or affiliated to CBOs. I likewise draw mainly on my research on this category of practitioners who are mainly working with post-test clubs or theatre associations. The post-test groups comprise people who have tested for HIV/AIDS and, irrespective of their status, have formed communities to support one another through joint activities such as pooling together to undertake small-scale business to economically support the members, reduce stigmatization, and advance positive living by having both HIV positive and those not (yet) seropositive associating. The other key activity of the post-test clubs is the use of theatre for education and sensitization of communities about AIDS. These clubs are mainly supported by local and international development organizations. One organization that has been prominent in this HIV/AIDS theatre support initiative is Plan International. The above are some of the contexts of work in theatre and HIV/AIDS that I draw on in discussing the nature of the space that applied theatre is negotiating. I will focus on highlighting the challenges.

A Brief Background to HIV/AIDS and Theatre Initiatives in Uganda

This discussion will focus on the challenges that applied theatre faces in the contexts of initiatives done in partnership with some CBOs. What is presented is not meant to be a depiction of the situation discussed as representative of the whole of HIV/AIDS theatre practice in Uganda. There are a number of initiatives that have delivered with significant effect and whose praxis in collaboration with theatre has produced works that are systematic and comparatively more effective. Research highlighting such positive work has been discussed widely.[3]

---

[3] See, for example, Marion Frank, *AIDS-Education Through Theatre: Case Studies from Uganda* (Bayreuth: Bayreuth African Studies, 1995); Rose Mbowa, "Theatre for Development: Empowering Ugandans to transform their condition," in *Developing Uganda*, ed. Holger Bernt Hansen & Michael Twaddle (Oxford: James Currey, 1998): 261–67; Patrick Mangeni, "Change in two hours: A theatre for development workshop with high school students in Kampala," and Patrick Mangeni, "A Theatrical Alternative for Child Survival: The Experience of School Health Drama in Uganda"; Carol Sicherman, "Drama and AIDS Education in Uganda: an interview with Rose

One of the post-Idi Amin developments Uganda has been known for is an open policy on the subject of HIV/AIDS education. In the 1980s, the Yoweri Museveni government acknowledged the scourge as a human and development hazard that called for mass action. Among the strategies adopted was the use of theatre for mass sensitization and mobilization. The focus of this campaign was on the factors and contexts of the HIV/AIDS spread. As I indicate above, the MoH, MoES, that of Information and Broadcasting (MoIB), and UNICEF were the most instrumental partners collaborating with theatre[4] The strategies were framed within the structures of the annual schools' Music, Dance and Drama Festivals. The schools, with their numerical strength, were chosen as sites for this campaign because they provided an army of learners and educators. As the more vulnerable and least infected group, children were conceptualized as a 'Window of Hope'. The strategy for securing and safeguarding this 'Window of Hope' included focusing on messages of: awareness-creation, the nature of AIDS and channels of infection, prevention strategies, supporting those infected and affected, and living positively with AIDS.

In terms of the state of AIDS awareness in Uganda, statistics indicate an 80% awareness of HIV/AIDS and how it is transmitted. This can be attributed to, among other factors, to the policy of mass education and other strategies that, for example, require schools to regularly address school children on HIV/AIDS; CBO-based development initiatives and associations that have informed its membership and developed publicity, information, and edutainment strategies and help those who are infected to access support and education on HIV/AIDS. The churches have also participated through music and competitive theatre organized for their communities and congregations.

The involvement of government through theatre has been mainly at the level of education and sensitization. For audiences outside the schools and communities around the school, the initiatives have involved governmental organizations partnering with theatre groups. A notable example was the production *Ndiwulira* by a popular urban-theatre group, Bakayimbira Dramactors, which was supported by the MoH and performed in stadiums and open grounds. This phase gave way to partnerships between individual theatre

---

Mbowa," in *History and Theatre in Africa*, ed. Yvette Hutchinson & Eckhard Breitinger (Bayreuth: Bayreuth African Studies 50, 2000): 109–18.

[4] Mangeni, "A Theatrical Alternative for Child Survival: The Experience of School Health Drama in Uganda"; Sicherman, "Drama and AIDS Education in Uganda: an interview with Rose Mbowa"; Frank, *AIDS-Education Through Theatre.*

practitioners/facilitators, consultancies of mostly two or one persons using theatre strategies for behavioural change to combat HIV/AIDS. This phase has been characterized by initiatives originated by local and international development organizations working in partnership with individuals/ consultancies at various levels to sensitize vulnerable communities on specific issues considered as exacerbating HIV/AIDS.

These partnership activities have been in critical development areas including gender, training theatre groups in the skills of playmaking and performance for AIDS education, and working with those who have associated as infected or affected members of post-test clubs. Theatre has, in these contexts, been used to build community, provide space for exploring HIV/AIDS, and broach issues that relate to development and for community education. In this latter case, the practice is partly premised on the notion that, owing to the saturation of AIDS messages, the use of the infected or affected as communicators of HIV/AIDS could be more effective and may increase audience identification with the message and subsequently education. It is these later phases and contexts of practice that I will draw on to discuss the nature of the space in which applied theatre is operating and negotiating and to reflect on the nature and challenges this space presents for applied-theatre praxis in general and HIV/AIDS in particular.

HIV/AIDS information fatigue exists, a situation that borders on breeding complacency and has partly been advanced to explain the increasing infection rates, especially among youth and married people. The theatre space is also characterized by the challenge of attendance and audience retention. Facilitators have reported audiences departing after watching the initial mobilization dance/performance. They are drawn by dance as entertainment.[5] Similarly, the entry of ARVs and their capacity to prolong life has given AIDS the face of a disease that is normal like other diseases. AIDS has been demystified, the fear of agonizing and early death minimized. This has been partly attributed to the medicines prolonging people's lives. ARVs have thus 'complicated' and made less obvious the practice of identifying the HIV-infected through their physical state. This has complicated the Applied-Theatre space. More 'topical' development challenges such as gender and poverty eradication have assumed prominence in development initiatives, leading a number of development organizations and government initiatives to focus on these concepts to structure development interventions. This has provided opportu-

[5] Julius Kyakuwa, personal communication, February, 2004.

nities to structure theatre initiatives to explore how these concepts relate and interface with HIV/AIDS.[6]

The Nature of the Space in Which Applied Theatre is Situated

In this discussion, I conceptualize space in terms of the factors, practices, and attitudes that characterize the environment in which applied theatre is operating. The discussion will consider the nature of this environment and how it informs and mediates the practice of and potential for applied theatre. The nature of this environment in which applied theatre is situated impacts on, defines, and mediates in the practice of applied-theatre research as a strategy for generating understanding and as a pretext for the application of these understandings to inform practice and advance change in society.

The nature of the mediating space in applied theatre is a contested site with overarching interests, values, and priorities. The different players in applied-theatre practice in Uganda attach and conceive varying meanings to this space and come with different values; these understandings inform perceptions of and approaches into the use of the space. These competing value systems then intersect to impact on the practice of and research in applied theatre. By seeking to contribute to this discussion by highlighting the nature of the space in which applied-theatre practice is situated, I hope to directly or indirectly facilitate reflection on what such a context may mean for applied-theatre initiatives in the context of HIV/AIDS education, not only in Uganda but perhaps, too, in Africa as a whole or even beyond.

Self-Interest and Nepotism

A variety of elements define the space in which applied theatre operates. The economics and the politics of the spaces inform the theatre environment and interrelate with issues of perception and values. One highlighted challenge to the practice of and capacity for theatre as empowerment and development has been the use of theatre by CBOs and facilitators primarily as a means of self-development – see Ahmed Sayed's "Wishing for a World without 'Theatre

---

[6] Baron Oron, personal communication, 25 January 2010.

for Development',"[7] on how some CBOs in Bangladesh have exploited the theatre space for their own economic interests. Sayed's argument provides a commentary on related experiences and the associated challenges with reference to practices by some CBOs in Uganda and Theatre for Development facilitators.

In Uganda, the more dominant scenario is of theatre practitioners (mostly with backgrounds in mainstream theatre practice) engaging in applied theatre only occasionally. In the case of applied-theatre practice, most engagement has been mainly supported by local development organizations that have HIV/AIDS education on their agenda. These organizations depend on international donors/aid organizations for the funding of their programmes. In most cases, their budgets are fully funded by the international donor bodies. In general, the practical procedures – from partner identification, through project execution and evaluation, to reporting – differ between the international NGOs and local CBOs.

The selection criteria cited have varied, and included qualifications in project planning and development, and skills in development communication and a background in music, dance, and drama. But very often, when it comes to skills that are required to execute the project, one notices gaps in knowledge of the practice and capacity of applied theatre. There is a tendency not to clarify the objectives of the programme and the criteria to assess performance or the impact of the programmes. This leaves a lot of room for improvisation by the facilitators. The measurement of and evaluation of the projects thus becomes problematic if they lack clear reference points. I will discuss later how this translates into challenges for reporting on any project's performance, and on evaluating it and researching the experience.

The conduct of applied theatre is defined by competition. I have found this space very competitive, and winning has, in a number of instances, nothing to do with merit. This element mediates in the strategies and operations that the artists and the organizations adopt in the conduct of their applied-theatre work. At times it presents as essentially a business space – a survival space. And how may this manifest as a challenge for interventions relating to HIV/AIDS or applied theatre in general? The process of bidding for applied-theatre work, mostly with CBOs, is complex: 'technical know-who', as the

[7] See Ahmed Sayed, "Wishing for a World without 'Theatre for Development': Demystifying the case of Bangladesh," *Research in Drama Education* 7.2 (2002): 207–19.

practice of influence-peddling has been known, is often a factor, particularly so when dealing with CBOs. A high degree of protectiveness defines and permeates this space. Artists and practitioners have tended to jealously 'protect' information on opportunities for applied-theatre work they source. The sources are often friends or accomplices and even relatives working with or knowing someone working with such an organization. In interviews with applied-theatre facilitators in 2004, four of five respondents indicated that, for a number of projects they had been engaged with, they had secured these contracts with the assistance of a relative, a friend, the programme officer of the contracting CBO, or someone who had a connection with the individual(s) charged with or having influence on the selection process. The fifth respondent, a more established practitioner, also acknowledged that 'technical know-who' was often a significant factor when sourcing applied-theatre contracts in partnership with CBOs. Other practitioners have acknowledged this but have seen it differently, highlighting the positive aspects of it as well:

> One thing that needs to be clear is that contacts are very important. It's a great thing to have contacts and yes some of these things are through contacts. In my case [...] my first engagement, Professor Rutruba [who engaged me] knew me at a personal level and he was a relative. So that exposed me. And [in] many other places people know there is so and so [and] I can work with him.[8]

However, whereas getting to learn of such tasks through an 'insider' need not necessarily be a problem, when such notification is made with intentions to favour (as is usually the case), to influence and also limit access to information to a selected few, that becomes a problem. And practitioners have acknowledged this:

> The recruiting agency can be biased and may want somebody who dances to their tune, they may want somebody they know and especially if it [the contracting partner] is local: If we [CBOs] are the ones. These local organizations, they tend to go for someone who is cheaper or somebody they know. And if you have [are dealing with] an organization like that, that does not have the morals, that can happen, they will get somebody who they know who they can eat the money with.[9]

---

[8] Oron, personal communication, 25 January, 2010.

[9] Oron, personal communication, 25 January 2010.

This practice is a challenge to the capacity of theatre processes, as it limits transparency, communication, and the potential of theatre to engage the most qualified person or the most effective/persuasive programme that could have been considered, were the processes more transparent. Other facilitators explained the 'protectiveness' in terms of the 'on-and-off, once-in-a-long-time' nature of applied-theatre opportunities (anonymous interviewees, February 2004 and 2009) – that, because it is usually a one-off project, an applied-theatre project presents an opportunity for income. And when such projects are short-term, they are closely sought, guarded, and compromised. One facilitator who requested anonymity observed:

> I have worked with them [names CBO] since 1998. Somebody designs the project because he is going to benefit out of it. So the objectives of the projects might be there but first of all he is looking at how he is going to benefit out of it. So many of these projects you can see [referring to project reports on the shelves] many of them we have not even had the supervision from the people that have given us these projects. Last year we had a very big project: 9 drama groups we were training. That was a big project. But I want to tell you that not a single person came to visit us. They only based [their assessment] on our reports. We could have even sat in our offices, written out that report and handed it to them. So if you ask me whether I have had an opportunity [for follow-up], really I have not had.[10]

The nature of engagement for the artists has been to facilitate at applied-theatre workshops and to prepare plays on HIV/AIDS as written sensitization dramas; alternatively, they have worked with selected theatre groups to develop dramas that are performed in the community. They are hired and paid for facilitation. Facilitators therefore often value training opportunities differently. Even for those employed in government institutions, such contracts and engagement are often valued, too, in terms of how they offset the living wage. With theatre work doubling as a side or occasional income source, I have observed a tendency among practitioners and their 'informers' in the contracting organization to compromise the process. In one case in 2004, I experienced a situation where bids to develop sensitization drama on reproductive health and HIV/AIDS were called. I entered the competition and my synopsis was selected and we signed the agreement to write the script. Shortly after, I was requested not to develop the script, because someone else had

[10] Anonymous interview, March 2003.

won the bid. I was informed that a decision had been made at a higher level. I was asked to accept compensation. This was an international organization, although the project officers I dealt with were predominantly local. It came to pass that the artist who 'won' the bid was known to the officer, who, it was claimed, had reversed the decision. Other facilitators have also observed this:

> But it is not only in TfD, it is everywhere. Whether it is in building houses… it is everywhere. It is a structural problem in local organizations. […] So these small local organizations don't have good morals. But I again believe where there is a mix of people recruiting; where you have an American, a British, a Kenyan there tends to be more integrity in the selection of people. I have also encountered situations where people want to give you a job and you give them something later.[11]

Similarly, in a situation where mainstream theatre work does not guarantee a living wage for the practitioner, applied theatre has become one of those alternative catchphrases and the ideal specialization (the other being film) that many theatre artists have adopted or claimed.

When the space is defined by protectiveness, it also presents challenges in accessing information to gain understanding of the situation, practices, and experiences of such theatre initiatives. Information is often managed very carefully, to the extent that the researcher is not likely to access such information, if it is imparted at all. While doing research on this subject in 2004, I tended to elicit responses from and access records from my former students rather than from people who were not. The information provided tended to be in the form of photographs of workshops. Information in the form of recordings and reports was not easily accessed, although there was evidence that they were available.

Survival and Accountability

'Survival' interests have also mediated in the level, nature, and focus of the reports and performance narratives that these experiences/practitioners have developed as records of their work. Of the about twenty workshops and performance reports that I accessed during research in 2004, more than half were narratives of 'success'. They emphasized the justification for applied-theatre

---

[11] Oron, personal communication, 25 January 2010.

workshops, which account they backed with testimonies from participants' 'voices'. The reports outlined the process, including programmes for the workshop and concluding with appendices of the area's political leaders highlighting the transformative experiences through theatre and 'doing an Oliver twist' – asking for more. To attribute the unavailability of records to 'protectiveness' would blur other features that define and explain this space. Lack of (systematic) documentation is partly a cultural problem – unless systematic and guided reporting procedures are provided, a number of facilitators will focus on storytelling and oral narrative. A number of facilitators come from mainstream theatre, which is of a storytelling and improvisatory nature. This is a feature that has been typified as a traditional African element,[12] but it also constitutes a problem when you work with or expect more structured narratives of processes. Generally, there is a considerable challenge with regard to documentation and record-keeping. This is partly attributed to failures by CBOs to have clear programme-management procedures.

> The NGOs have very good objectives, but people on the ground who are implementing do not have those objectives. Ok they are supposed to do these things but at the end of the day, it's money they are looking for. You know this is Uganda. Somebody will give you a project and will need a kickback-nfunirawa?[13]

It is a national problem that is not limited to applied-theatre practice. One way to address part of this challenge is for anyone researching this process to get a better understanding of the experiences by observing the recording of the process of production or workshops. The protectiveness of practitioners can also be explained by their vulnerability to likely exposure. This poses ethical challenges. I observed, in researching four projects that a consultancy had carried out with a number of post-test groups they were contracted to train, that they were basically using the same play and passing it off as a different play on subsequent projects with the same or other local development organizations/partners. There has been evidence of facilitators recycling the content or plays for different audiences, as discussed above. In three of the cases I observed in 1996 and four in 2003–2006, the facilitators only changed the title of the play; the plot was basically the same.

[12] See Oga S. Abah, "Perspectives in Popular Theatre: Orality as a Definition of New Realities," in *Performance in Africa: Intercultural Perspectives*, ed. Eckhard Breitinger (Bayreuth, Bayreuth African Studies 31, 2003): 79–100.

[13] Anonymous, personal communication, February 2004.

In contexts where applied-theatre work is valued as an opportunity to earn, then other variables are negotiated to ensure job security and sustainability. What is emerging in some contexts is the formation of CBOs and applied-theatre consultancies when a bid is announced. This scenario perhaps explains a common phenomenon of artists starting organizations/consultancies for every contract advertised. This is not limited to applied-theatre artists. The reader who is familiar with contract/bidding business corruption narratives in Uganda will recall the Global Fund saga where money intended for HIV/AIDS programmes was swindled. Funds released to facilitate an investigation of another related scandal were also swindled. In the Global Fund instance, the commission of inquiry unearthed instances of organizations that were set up as fronts for sourcing the Global Fund, often fraudulently. In the case of applied theatre, a consultant/facilitator talked of an applied-theatre partner registering two organizations but undertaking similar applied-theatre activities. In the same period, the same partner also registered a third organization with this facilitator as a co-director. The objectives of the three organizations were similar. While this is not the norm, it is often the case where shareholders are suspicious of their partners or where they have differing views on how to allocate and share resources. Some artists have explained this as insecurity and mistrust, as discussed below. In other cases, the registering of more than one organization while concurrently partnering with another consultant enabled one to undertake projects unnoticed by the partner.

The most common groupings and/or associations were of husband and wife or parent and child registering a theatre-for-development organization. Wives have in some cases been sent to school or perhaps chosen carefully or provided with the necessary training to boost their skills-base in anticipation of such applied-theatre associations. There have been also cases of spouses or children learning on the job.

This is not to say that husbands and wives cannot effectively execute applied-theatre projects. A number of successful businesses have been founded and run on a family and heritage basis and they have performed successfully. Such affinities have at times acted as sources of cohesion. Filial and kinship connections and those based on marriage and related forms of intimate filiation can at times be reinforcing in some work settings.[14] However, this presents challenges when the wife is too often the treasurer. In a number of instances, co-directors in such organizations have been suspicious and

[14] Oron, interview, 25 January 2010.

some have complained of lack of transparency. This has been one cause of splits in membership of theatre-for-development organizations and has subsequently led to founding of new consultancies/CBOs.[15] This scenario impacts variously on the capacity of the theatre space. Organizations that experience this situation of splits are limited in their capacity to develop structures for sustainability.

This situation also creates the challenge of having aesthetic critical distance in praxis, of drawing the line between family and work. In such cases, the power and gender interplays have very often compromised work. One respondent explained that he ceased working with a colleague partly because she had drawn her child into the programme, was fretting about the child all the time, and also believed the child's report on facilitation in contrast to the co-facilitator's perception of the child's actual performance, ultimately at the expense of the work. In another case, one facilitator had to quit a consultancy after the partner passed away. He could not continue with the consultancy, because, according to him, it meant that the late partner's shares "were supposed to be inherited by his family [...] who didn't have any knowledge as far as theatre was concerned." He was not prepared to share proceeds, because the family would not be making any contribution to the running of the consultancy. This director left the consultancy and founded one with his wife as a co-director.[16]

So, when a local theatre organization is founded on a premise of business and protectionism and if a couple claim it as their own, how can one negotiate these spaces among individuals and organizations intended to facilitate change? How might filial relationship exert an influence on endeavours to develop structures that are sustainable? And how might such an interested party respond to the researcher in the face of 'sharing family experiences'. How else can we triangulate to authenticate their claims? I have experienced reluctance on the part of a number of facilitators to share experiences of practice when they thought that such sharing would expose them to scrutiny.

The other observable feature of groups or 'consultancies' geared towards 'survival' is lack of structures. Often formed to execute an 'advertised' applied-theatre task, they dissolve when that need is met. This ephemeral and circumstantial nature of such organizations raises challenges for research in particular. And this relates to their capacity to observe, generate, and collect data or develop records of their work, as discussed above. Records have not

---

[15] Martin Kintu, interview, February 2004.

[16] Anonymous, personal communication, February 2004.

been a feature of interest among practitioners and contracting local development partners:

> They don't really do things as they are supposed to be done. That is why you see that follow-ups are not done. Whereas [...] the country office think people [programme officers] are doing the right thing, they don't. [...] They have always depended on reports and once you give them reports, that is it. And I want to tell you that they may not even read these reports. They don't. [We do reports] because you have to attach a report in order to make your claim.[17]

Oron confirmed this:

> It is very difficult to put you to account for the time and the money because they are guilty they took part of the money. Two; because you don't have professional supervision, you will not feel like doing a very good job. You will not do the difficult tasks in TfD especially in engaging the people in dialogue and following the processes through and through. It will affect the quality and you will not write a good report. Nobody is going to write a good report about an activity that has not been followed up, an activity that is not bringing results.[18]

This raises subsequent challenges for the researcher who might be interested in accessing the record of the experience to facilitate understanding the nature of the impact of the programmes as HIV/AIDS intervention. Thus, when projects are valued differently by the facilitators and CBOs this raises questions about the nature and reliability of the narratives of theatre praxis that researchers seek to access. A number of records I observed were mainly reports of plot summaries (as discussed above). The nature of record-keeping was often by memory. While engaged in research with consultancies that were involved with performing groups to advance positive living and HIV/AIDS awareness in Luwero, I noted that more than half of the twenty-six reports I accessed had used the same template: plot narrative, mammoth community attendance and commendations and memoranda from the local leaders asking for more shows due to public demand. It came to my understanding that, in such cases, some of the reports are fashioned in collaboration between project coordinators and the consultants/facilitators. This is normally done to use such reports as supporting evidence that the project was successful and useful to the community. This in turn is fashioned to enable continued sup-

---

[17] Anonymous, personal communication, February 2004.

[18] Personal communication, 25 January 2010.

port/funding of programmes. Both facilitators and project coordinators operating under this arrangement partly value and manage the reporting and evaluation process of the project as opportunities to get further support (income). The question, therefore, is: How else might one gain access to this space in order to engage with it, to learn andlor enable understanding of the performance of HIV/AIDS processes and initiatives?

Researching such experiences then becomes problematic. Very often, some 'consultants' did not recall well what project took place where and when. When the task demands comprehensive reporting, this is when you encounter this challenge.

Researching the Space

In the case of the research I conducted, one research strategy/tool that was helpful in recapturing the experiences was drawing from the scanty project reports as prompts and pretexts for developing interview guides. The interview method, especially in the form of focused group discussions, proved to be a useful research strategy for gaining greater understanding and details on the theatre experience. But the focus-group strategy for data collection was more appropriate when one needed information and details on the theatre experiences of particular workshops or production performance experiences and where only plot outlines as data were available. The focus-group discussion method was also helpful in recollecting experiences in post-production discussions or information on how the facilitators attempted to negotiate where their audiences were apathetic towards HIV/AIDS education. Individual interviews were more appropriate when seeking understanding of how facilitators negotiated the competitive applied-theatre space.

Except for graduates of Makerere University's department of Music, Dance and Drama of the early 1990s, most other practitioners had not received formal education in the theory and practice of applied theatre. Against such a background, AIDS drama has been predominantly sensitization. According to Oron,

> The TfD we have is the TfD we learnt at school and then we went to the field … up to now we don't have a curricular. The department could be having a curricular for training the students but we do not have a book that we can give out to people… in most cases TfD tends

> to vary from person to person depending on how she has used it before and these other skills.[19]

Post-production discussions, where they have been conducted, have tended to focus more on explicating the audiences' understanding of the plot.[20] Similarly, the time provided for reflection on the performance has often been limited and the facilitators have exhibited a need for training in facilitation skills. This need was more pronounced where the consultants were operating in contexts where, for instance, plays on HIV/AIDS were performed by post-test groups to communities. Where communities have been performed to by individuals that have tested for HIV/AIDS and where some are visibly sick, the audience has been challenged in negotiating between the drama and the life of the individuals. Appropriate facilitation skills are needed to focus the post-production reflection phase on the issues raised or represented in the drama. Secondly, there is a need for skills to manage the process so that the actors are protected, as some questions from the audiences have tended to be personal, thereby risking stigmatization for the performer. In all the cases we discussed there were no qualified counsellors as a support mechanism, given the psychological implications and therapeutic support-needs that might arise from the theatre process. On the whole, however, participation by the community in these HIV/AIDS projects was limited to members taking part in mobilization performances at the beginning and at the end of the show. Because of the lack of strategies for qualitative participation, the retention of the audience is often a challenge.

This challenge is not only as a result of strategic limitations in planning but partly due to audience fatigue with the HIV/AIDS subject and the sensitization focus of communication. Some facilitators have responded to this challenge by developing strategies to counter it and to attract and retain audiences. These have included the use of public address systems playing recorded music of popular local musicians such as Jose Chameleon and Bobi Wine. They have also drawn on and used popular traditional dance rhythms such as the key Kiganda dance motif of Bakisimba-Nankasa-Muwogoala drum rhythms.[21] The Gisu Kadodi rhythms for processional dance have been

[19] Personal communication, 25 January 2010.

[20] Kintu, personal communication, February 2004.

[21] Kyakuwa, personal communication, March 2004.

effective in drawing in communities.[22] The latter rhythm is a popular circumcision motif, thus raising the expectation of seeing circumcision initiates and captivating pelvic gyrations and the animated waist-movements from dancers moving suggestively on staccato beats. Through announcements during mobilization and the beginning of the show, the organizers and facilitators promise a mega-happening at the end as a way to retain the audience.[23]

A significant number of communities we have worked with in HIV/AIDS drama interventions with CBOs have tended to exhibit more interest if applied-theatre processes help to advance their daily survival needs. These communities have been more supportive of initiatives that will improve their lives; in particular, they will answer questions on food, shelter, fees, capital for business, and medicines for those needing ARVs. I have registered a low level of interest from participants when attempting to privilege research or understanding. Part of the problem has been that applied theatre has been fashioned as a form that 'solves' people's problems; as a quick-fix panacea. Whereas applied-theatre initiatives that are of a workshop nature, involving cyclic process aimed at enhancing understanding, are received more positively, in academic contexts, in communities, such workshops have generally been received with reluctance.

Thus, in communities where people are poor and are preoccupied more with survival, theatre practice that seeks to privilege processes of conscientization without, for instance, addressing issues of pit latrines are treated as luxuries. In such locations, theatre is valued if it directly contributes food to the table. And because of low participation, where mostly men attend, the narratives that emerge have tended to be less representative. Men will tend not to want to participate unless there is some form of remuneration. When I have worked with post-test groups, narratives that sought to focus on AIDS directly were not prioritized except if they were linked to the daily struggles of survival. In the case of participation, men have been less inclined to seek membership in the theatre process of post-test organizations. For example, a post-test group I worked with in Mulago had a registered membership of twenty-

---

[22] Patrick Mangeni, "Negotiating Learning Contexts: Some Experiences of Culture, Power and Gender in Working with Multi-Cultural Communities through Theatre for Development," in *Universal Mosaic of Drama and Theatre:The IDEA 2004 Dialogues*, ed. Laura McCammon & Debra McLauchlan (Toronto: IDEA Publications, 2006): 233–43.

[23] Kintu, personal communication, February 2004.

four women as against four men, in instances where the process gave participants the opportunity to choose or identify and prioritize issues. Martin Kintu of Theatre Partners observed the same tendency of men being disinclined to participate. There is also a tendency not to privilege HIV/AIDS as the subject for dramatic explorations. For instance, in the eight weeks of workshops on HIV/AIDS that I conducted in Mulago in 2004, HIV/AIDS was not identified as a key issue except if it was constructed to lead to an intervention in their situation such as the care and education of AIDS orphans. This underscores the importance of HIV/AIDS theatre processes being contextualized and practised in a more holistic context. This is captured by Oron when he explains his experience of negotiating this limitation:

> For me I enhance TfD with the skills I get from some packages like stepping stones… so you find that you are drawing from a number of sources…other packages have helped me to appreciate the use of TfD better. […] if you are looking at TfD and HIV you are looking at behavioral change communication. We are looking at improving our knowledge. Changing our attitudes to change from negative to positive and also our practices… so when someone is able to combine these skills in TfD and knowledge from programming; looking at behavioral change, looking at community advocacy, looking at it from that perspective, you are able to become a stronger person, because all these skills which you get help to shape us up.[24]

This challenge relates to and also highlights poverty as a feature that informs and intervenes in this space. The majority of participants in theatre-and-HIV/AIDS programmes have thus been members of or audiences from impoverished environments living in suburbs and slums of the urban areas. Where the groups are in outlying rural or semi-urban districts, theatre interventions have used theatre groups to disseminate information and work with the communities. In either of these categories of population, they do not have salaried employment. In the case of the urban areas, they engage in petty (roadside) trade as market vendors, hawkers, or housewives. Those belonging to post-test clubs enter applied-theatre initiatives and external projects with the background of being supported by CBOs. Such support, in the case of the HIV-infected includes provision of ARVs, food supplements, and in some cases foodstuffs. This background has often turned into expectations of support from any outsider. This challenge of expectations is informed by the sub-

---

[24] Personal communication, 25 January 2010.

text of poverty, as intimated above. applied theatre thus enters poor space and, where this has occurred, processes aimed at gaining understanding through workshop and research are at times seen as not responding to the basic necessities of the community. Otherwise outcomes of such processes are often seen as benefitting the researcher. For instance, in 2004, I went to Kampala City Council Health centre in Kawempe division, where a number of post-test groups were assembled that day for counselling, food, and medical support. I was seeking a group to conduct workshops with. I was confronted with a question that is not unusual in Uganda, *nfunira wa?* meaning 'what do I gain from it?' This was from an all-men's group. Research or processes aimed at achieving understanding, whether by researchers or for participants, is often perceived as the researcher's agenda. Thus, unless funded, independent research is deeply influenced by poverty.

Like the CBOs which need positive reports to continue getting donor support, these participants become protective of the process whereby they are remunerated. In one such workshop in Mulago in 2004, group leaders attempted to discipline a participant who expressed views that were interpreted by fellow participants as threatening the continuity of the project. Interestingly, the participant's concern was whether I would pay them allowances for days that we had initially planned for workshops but on which we were not able to work. He expected 'transport' money, although he lived within walking distance. With poverty intervening in the theatre space, this raises questions about the reliability of data if participants valued the process primarily as contributing to their livelihood and sustenance. Groups and participants who were housewives and dependent on their husbands, and those on ARV, tended to be more 'compliant' and sensitive to views and actions that were interpreted as likely to undermine the continuation of opportunities that such applied-theatre processes offered. In such circumstances, survival is a priority over intervention in HIV/AIDS. As someone put it, 'Hunger will kill you today, but AIDS takes a longer time'.

Another challenge is that of patronage, which often takes the form of a project officer of the contracting CBO participating in the selection process. S/he may front a company of someone they have an 'understanding' with. This understanding often involves commissions which are at times paid up-front by the 'bidder' or may be retained at the time of payment for services. In some cases programme/project officers from the contracting CBO are (co)-directors of or have shares/interest in the bidding company. Some of these organizations have been founded specifically for these purposes. Where shareholding interest has not been legally registered, the programme officer may retain, or is advanced, his/her quota of payments being remitted. The facilitator/consultant pays a percentage. In some cases the Programme officer assists the bidder who agrees on giving the highest commission. This becomes more complicated especially where the process of applying for, winning, and processing the bid has more than one level of decision-making. In the latter case, and if they are compromised, the commission expected if not factored in the bid quote, as is often the case, leaves the person winning the bid with fewer resources with which to execute the programme. The way some consultancies have negotiated around this is to ask for supplementary budgets, which, if not inflated to meet the expected shortfall, end up as another opportunity for 'commissions'.

Where such cases have occurred, this culture of commissions, patronage, and interest has proved to be a huge challenge for applied-theatre projects in terms of planning resource allocation within the activity areas. It affects the reporting and above all the capacity for affected projects to realize the schedules. In one such case, money demanded as bribes was more than money allocated for the project. Often there is little, if anything, left for the work.

A facilitator I interviewed in 2006 talked about a theatre project on HIV/AIDS sensitization that was paid for but never took place:

> Actually with even [names CBO] we had stories [...] where people have been given projects and they have not done them and they have just sat on their desks to write reports. [...] it's a moral issue to receive money to work with AIDS people and you forge a report and get money. It is morally inappropriate. This is not only for theatre but other projects they [CBO] are trying to implement. There are certain things they have written on reports that they have supplied and they have not. [...] Drugs meant for AIDS patients have not been delivered.[25]

According to the informant, reports of this 'project' were prepared and presented to the organization, and the programme officer acknowledged the workshop as having taken place. While this may be the exception, and whereas a number of projects are being conducted through more transparent processes, this tendency cannot be dismissed as just as a one-off. It is symptomatic of the practice we call in Uganda 'supplying air', where you have 'briefcase organizations' colluding with those who are charged with the

[25] Anonymous, personal communication, February 2003.

responsibility to oversee execution of projects to pay themselves for work that was supposed to be done. This situation turns the applied-theatre space into a competitive, political, economic, and, at times, survival space where money and influence mediate in the processes for developing, executing, assessing, and evaluating applied-theatre experiences. Perhaps a 'good' side of such experiences is that they offer us an opportunity to reflect on how else this challenge can be negotiated. As Oron noted,

> where you are recruited because people want something from you or because they want to help you and not because of your skills, it will mean that you are not going to deliver … it means they are not getting the right quality and so that impacts on the work. […] It is very difficult to put you to account for the time and the money because they are guilty they took part of the money. Too, because you don't have professional supervision, you will not feel like doing a very good job. You will not do the difficult tasks in TfD especially in engaging the people in dialogue and following the processes through and through. It will affect the quality and you will not write a good report. Nobody is going to write a good report about an activity that has not been followed up, an activity that is not bringing results… and so it affects the programmes.[26]

Thus, to improve of the quality of reporting on applied-theatre projects to reflect the intended goals and how the project performed through theatre, the contracting CBOs will need to highlight the criteria for reporting. A number of local development organizations with which applied-theatre facilitators have worked do not provide these guidelines. This creates problems when facilitators are asked to provide reports or to do performance evaluations. In a number of cases, where I have been involved with CBOs, I and my teams have had to sit with programme officers of the contracting organizations to develop the assessment criteria. This has guided us in designing our methodology, intervention tools, and the measurement and evaluation of work.

Interestingly, in one case, when I proposed to the chief of the organization that he set up a forum for me to disseminate the findings arising from the project I had carried out with them, the executive asked for a four-page summary instead. This tendency is partly because the interest of most CBOs in applied theatre is to use it to sensitize or educate. It is the practice aspect that they are interested in. This latter component is what often defines their goals and

[26] Personal communication, 25 January 2010.

engagement with theatre. Often a number of CBOs will have conducted their baseline research. This is usually on the needs aspect – a needs assessment. Against such background, theatre is seen or valued as a means of realizing the answers to the problem identified: a tool of change and delivery.

Research in applied-theatre practice has been mainly championed by drama departments in the university as part of course requirements. Some of these academic practices have generated literature in the form of publications and research reports, as indicated above. The attainment of qualifications has been the end-point of a number of projects. The other category is the collaboration between academics at universities and CBOs. The level of engagement has been in terms of designing project-implementation strategies. This has included maintaining the project in the role of facilitator. When research is conducted, however, it is done so as an individual initiative, with the CBOs at times exhibiting minimal interest, as discussed above. Such a scenario then raises the question: How may such practice support change and development? The lack of interest in the research component of applied theatre by CBOs also suggests that research findings obtained from such projects may often not be widely disseminated, nor is it likely that any findings advocating improvement will be implemented. This attitude thus informs research strategy and execution.

Evaluation

Where guidelines are not provided, it has been problematic attempting to evaluate and research the performance of applied-theatre initiatives both in the area of HIV/AIDS and in other development areas. In some instances, politicians have tended to opportunistically fill this vacuum. They have exploited this gap in the performance space to gain political mileage and influence reporting; emphasizing elements that indicate good performance for them as politicians. A politician's performance is partly measured by his or her capacity to attract development projects. As indicated earlier in this discussion, a typical report is also followed by recommendations for more shows of the kind; the political leaders then say the programme was a success. Involvement of large numbers of the community in any project is also seen as an indicator of performance. The large numbers, real or imagined, are translated into a public demand. These challenges, which are created mainly by structural and operational weaknesses, create a vacuum that the local leaders exploit for personal political purposes.

As noted at the outset, CBOs have focused more on raising awareness through sensitization drama; this has been the terms of participation. CBOs provide raw data on AIDS and the dramatists translate this into dramatic messages. The challenge with such a method is that much is done, but there is limited space within the framework. Space provided is for narrative reports that are restricted to providing an overview. The focus of this report does not privilege the evaluation of the strategies of drama. It does not provide space for reflexivity and drawing new knowledge about their application. At the level of awareness-creation, using the numerical strength of the number of people attending as the measure of programme effectiveness or the number of venues performed becomes problematic. This is an aspect that a number of trainers and CBOs have clashed on as a success indicator. I must admit I often found it very frustrating trying to make sense of and gain understanding of the experience of a number of HIV/AIDS workshops that some consultancies conducted in the Buganda region from the late 1990s to the early 2000s. As this number-based assessment is a predominant feature of research-report narratives from practitioners who are the majority in the field, and without discounting other projects that are well executed, I am concerned about how else we might negotiate this challenge. It is a challenge also of educating the contracting partners. As Oron observes,

> Very few people still appreciate it. In many cases people will look at theatre as a tool just for community mobilization. Many people come and watch a drama and they go away. People at the project level, the NGOs don't know, they don't know how theatre for development works. These big people you see in offices here they just know that the message is relayed; people see it and then just go.[27]

We need to negotiate for qualitative evaluation of the process to be part of the applied-theatre space. If some CBOs do not value or emphasize comprehensive reporting back, while we should consider initiating and sharing experiences about the need and value of measurement and evaluation, we also need to consider alternative strategies of capturing data through, for instance, investing in facilities for and encouraging video recordings of applied-theatre and HIV/AIDS experiences. If some artists are primarily focusing on managing the politics of winning and sustaining themselves in the projects for their survival, it is important for us, where we have not yet done so, to explore how else we might negotiate this political environment for strategic space to

---

[27] Personal communication, 25 January 2010.

enable us capture the experience, in ways that will offer an opportunity for more representative knowledge and understanding. How else, then, might this space be negotiated?

Quality in the Applied-Theatre Space

The perception of applied theatre as culture and cultural expression has intervened in the effectiveness of applied theatre as sensitization and information dissemination. One challenge I have found is that communities have been brought to believe that applied theatre has the power to find solutions to challenges faced by individuals and communities, and, indeed, that it finds such solutions. At the Drama for Life conference of 2008, during a playback theatre workshop, I shared an experience of falling victim to this 'gospel' when I talked about a session I was facilitating in Uganda in the late 1990s. It had happened that an actor was performing her challenge and fear of being evicted from her accommodation for non-payment of rent. The enactment of the participant's problem, a dilemma she was facing in real life, was interrupted by her actual landlord. He had walked into the scene of enactment and demanded that the actor/tenant either pay up rent arrears or vacate the house. All of the participants, who identified with the situation, turned to me expectantly. Neither the applied-theatre process nor I and the other three facilitators could find any way of intervening to 'solve' the problem.

Thus, the idealization of the post-performance phase of the applied-theatre workshop process has, in some cases, generated reluctance to participate in AIDS-related initiatives through applied theatre except if they are tied to provision of support for the sick, as discussed above. But we all know applied theatre cannot answer many of the questions, let alone all of them. What is needed is a collaborative strategy with other disciplines and development initiatives. For instance, the value of applied theatre should be emphasized in its capacity to enhance participation and the understanding of issues, researching and raising awareness. For instance, the fields of medicine, community health, and psychology have shown a capacity to support the process of the community's physical and emotional challenges that intervene in their development. The practice of collaborative research initiatives has proved to be a key feature which applied theatre must embrace in its mission of HIV/AIDS education and social development.

There is a challenge to appreciating and understanding applied theatre as a field of practice and as a discipline. Whereas a number of artists draw on indigenous art forms, especially the aspect of spontaneity and improvisation for flexibility in the theatre process in order to allow the participants to tell and perform their stories, often this element of traditional African theatre performance has been oversimplified. Secondly, there is still a tendency on the part of some CBOs to reduce theatre to singing, dancing, and acting, revealing how some CBOs value theatre and what they expect from the process of applied theatre. This kind of understanding has compromised the quality of the theatre space. For instance, resources needed, such as time for executing projects and facilitating understanding of the experiences, have in most instances been limited. This perception has not provided optimum space for critical and informed practice and for the monitoring and evaluation of theatre practice. 'Naturally', the focus of documentation of such initiatives and collaboration has privileged plot narratives and audience attendance, as discussed above.

Another challenge concerns the expectations and perceptions of some of the practitioners about what they consider to be their training needs. There have been occasions on which some facilitators-trainees have wanted 'cookbook' packages on the applied-theatre process. This is a national problem that is not limited to the applied-theatre space. Educationists and critics of the education system in Uganda have expressed concern, especially at tertiary level, about the need to develop critical thinkers and problem-solvers rather than rote learners. Unfortunately, the system has produced a generation of students who do not seem to be interested in deeper questions. This raises concerns for the future of scholarship in applied theatre, given that it is in the universities that researchers in applied-theatre praxis are groomed.

A number of practitioners involved in applied-theatre work are there, perhaps, mainly because it is the 'in thing' that can bring quick(er) money. It is also not uncommon for artists who have participated in an applied-theatre workshop for the first time to 'pass' out and pose as experts. There has also been a tendency for students who have just graduated from theatre courses, at Makerere University in particular, to open up consultancies as experts. In other cases, artists who may not have formal training in applied theatre have started consultancies after working for a brief time with more senior facilitators. The effect, in a number of instances, has been to downgrade the applied-theatre process to messaging and poorly facilitated improvisations. The understanding is that applied theatre is about creating a play showing your problems and then to identify solutions. This is one area where intervention in the form of education and training of facilitators is much needed. In the skills area, facilitation is little understood. Most of us know the centrality of facilitation in the theatre process as empowerment. There is a need to appreciate facilitation in its entirety and the facilitator's capacity to influence the process to enhance understanding. Generally, there has in practice been an emphasis on the community's being able to participate in the applied-theatre process but less on the person enabling the process. Perception of drama as a simple affair of acting a situation affects engagement, criteria of evaluation, and the reporting system. This affects the quality of knowledge produced in applied theatre in AIDS education and intervention contexts.

Conclusion

I also wish to acknowledge the important point that most HIV/AIDS initiatives have been launched and executed by international NGOs supporting CBOs. They have also done this in collaboration with Government, as discussed above. The areas of focus in Uganda, for instance, have been on awareness-creation and behavioural change. Where theatre has been applied, it has been mainly as a tool of mass awareness through education campaigns. There has also been a focus on the inculcation of positive living. The focus in this space has been the individual. The form applied has been of advocacy. However, there is also a lack of will to invest meaningfully in culturally based processes. applied-theatre processes draw on culturally based forms of performance practice because of their capacity to communicate quickly and effectively, embodying as they do everyday artforms. This at times has led to a misconception and oversimplification of applied theatre as process by the CBOs and facilitators.

CBOs have not always supported investment in culture, particularly CBOs oriented towards gender and development. HIV interventions through theatre have tended to focus on the problematics of multiple sexual partners, prostitutes, unfaithful adults, and cross-generational sex. And although there is 80% awareness of the risk of unprotected sex as the key conduit for HIV infections, 80% (the majority young people) practice unprotected sex. When culture is interpreted as an impediment to gender equity, some initiatives that focus on culture have tended to do so in order to demonize culture instead of structuring the processes to enable the examination of customs and traditions to advance and highlight gender agendas. For instance, in some cases polygamy has often been over-emphasized as a leading cause of HIV/AIDS. And yet, as the 'anti sexual network' campaign has clearly identified, sexual networking is rife even in monogamous relations, let alone among young people and the unmarried. It is crucial that culture is not narrowly interpreted as some retrogressive indigenous practice but as that which is and defines us at a given moment – that which we must persistently interrogate without attempting to be culturally clever or patronizing. Unfortunately, polygamy has been narrowly linked with promiscuity and AIDS. It is a false premise, a reductionist way of seeing, a patronizing strand of cultural imperialism. If the challenge is AIDS, then the focus is perhaps sexual networks and not polygamy per se. Further, to focus on the traditional sites for infection in anti HIV/AIDS campaigns means leaving out those young sexually active children and especially sexually active youth who were born with HIV/AIDS.

When the post-test clubs, initiated and supported by HIV/AIDS-based organizations such as the AIDS Support Organization (TASO), the AIDS Information Centre (AIC), and CBOs such as Plan International, began establishing and supporting the post-test communities and used them in AIDS-awareness campaigns (theatre groups such as Bakayimbira Dramactors had been used in these crusades), the problem arose (also in some mainstream theatre groups) of audiences expecting the actors to live what they preach on stage. Unfortunately, many of the groups have lost their actors to HIV/AIDS. I recall that, when I was in Rakai District in 1988–89 working with theatre groups in a build-up to the National Youth Festivals in Kampala, many of the participants who had been selected from the groups were not able to make it to Kampala for the festivals because they had died of AIDS. Nor, in follow-up interviews in 2004, was I able to reach a number of participants from Mityana, Rakai, and Kampala districts. I was informed by a respondent[28] that these, too, had died of AIDS. In this regard, actors and theatre groups stand out distinctly, as their non-stage lives are open to public scrutiny. When they are infected with or affected by conditions such as AIDS, unlike all 'ordinary' persons, the public is more inclined to generalize their condition as a result of a sexually permissive lifestyle. So, when transmitters of AIDS messages are seen as vectors, this presents a challenge of using actors, outside the mainstream post-test clubs, in anti-AIDS Theatre initiatives. There are thus challenges for us as theatre artists negotiating between role and real-life experiences. Our audiences hold the mirror up to us. How might this inform our capacity to get our message across? And how else might we frame our practice to successfully negotiate the problematic area? Perhaps we need to make

[28] Interview with Joseph Walugembe, March 2004.

space in our practice to explore our place within these processes. Do we or, even, should we also put our lives within this space, or do we take the safe position of facilitator and researcher? And do we in our reports reflect on our experiences within the subjectivity of investigation or do we assume the safer distance of a participant observer?

WORKS CITED

Abah, Oga S. "Perspectives in Popular Theatre: Orality as a Definition of New Realities," in *Theatre and Performance in Africa: Intercultural Perspectives*, ed. Eckhard Breitinger (Bayreuth: Bayreuth African Studies, 2003): 79–100.

Frank, Marion. *AIDS-Education Through Theatre: Case Studies from Uganda* (Bayreuth: Bayreuth African Studies, 1995).

Mangeni, Patrick. "Change in two hours: A theatre for development workshop with high school students in Kampala," *Researching Drama in Education Journal* 3.1 (1998): 93–96.

——. "Negotiating Learning Contexts: Some Experiences of Culture, Power and Gender in Working with Multi-Cultural Communities through Theatre for Development," in *Universal Mosaic of Drama and Theatre: The IDEA 2004 Dialogues*, ed. Laura McCammon & Debra McLauchlan (Toronto: IDEA Publications, 2006): 233–43.

——. "A Theatrical Alternative for Child Survival: The Experience of School Health Drama in Uganda," in *Drama, Culture and Empowerment*, ed. John O'Toole & Kate Donelan (Brisbane: IDEA Publications, 1996): 77–85.

Mbowa, Rose. "Theatre for Development: Empowering Ugandans to transform their condition," in *Developing Uganda*, ed. Holga Bernt Hansen & Michael Twaddle (Oxford: James Currey, 1998): 261–70.

Sayed, Ahmed S. "Wishing for a World without 'Theatre for Development': Demystifying the case of Bangladesh," *Research in Drama Education* 7.2 (2002): 207–19.

Sicherman, Carol. "Drama and AIDS Education in Uganda: an interview with Rose Mbowa," in *History and Theatre in Africa*, ed. Yvette Hutchinson & Eckhard Breitinger (Bayreuth: Bayreuth African Studies 50, 2000): 109–18.

⌘

DAVID KERR

HIV Communication

Global Emergencies, Media Templates, and African Communities (A Personal Journey)

I THINK THE BEST WAY FOR ME TO DISCUSS MEDIA in relation to training of drama practitioners in the field of HIV/AIDS is to explain some of my own experiences and shifting attitudes in the field of both face-to-face and mediated communication. These changes have affected not only my own pedagogy over the years but also that of many colleagues.

My first major experience of drama teaching in Africa was in fact a media product, making, between 1971 and 1973 at the University of Malawi, a short, 16mm black-and-white film based on a Malawian folk-tale. The experience taught me the amazing ability of Malawians (both students and ordinary villagers) to become creatively involved in cooperative filmmaking. The other lesson, due to some scary political interference from the President's Office, was how the public nature of media magnified the dangers of censorship.[1] Despite continuing media activities, radio drama, and features in Malawi, television drama in Zambia, video in Botswana, and print production of magazines in all three countries, my main focus tended towards live stage drama and street theatre, owing to its lower profile and much more flexible working methods.

---

[1] David Kerr, *Dance, Media Entertainment & Popular Theatre in South East Africa* (Bayreuth: Bayreuth African Studies 43, 1996): 175–76; Mufunanji Magalasi, "Stage Drama in Independent Malawi: 1980 to 2002" (doctoral dissertation, University of Malawi, Zomba 2006): 45.

From the late 1970s in Zambia and the early 1980s in Malawi, I began to conceptualize, and possibly romanticize the Southern African village audience as a participatory community, which could create for itself a discursive space, more democratic than the public discourse of both national and local politics.

In the struggle to achieve such a space, my colleagues and I tended to revert to a very simplistic ethical framework; we and the ordinary workers and peasants we worked with were the 'good guys', the imperialists and the neo-colonialists were the 'bad guys'. Although we were astute enough to realize the porous nature of this division, the binary categories crept into much of our strategizing, activism, and even aesthetics. In one essay, the Zimbabwean theatre activist Stephen Chifunyise and I borrowed from Walter Benjamin's aesthetic contrasts between Aristotelian and Epic Theatre to create similar lists pointing out the difference between imported, neo-colonialist theatre forms and popular African theatre.[2]

My attitude to mediated forms of drama had a similar simplistic division. Vestiges of those binaries can be found in my book *African Popular Theatre*, where I borrow, from the Filipino theatre group PETA, the concept of micro-media (mostly small-scale face-to-face drama) and macro-media, large-scale media productions usually from multi-national media corporations.[3] Although I didn't provide any politico-aesthetic lists in the book, I did make them with my students in seminars on the following lines.

MACRO-MEDIA DRAMA	MICRO-COMMUNITY THEATRE
Multi-national media corporations	Small-scale production companies
Huge budgets	Small, self-sufficient funding
Synergies built into marketing strategies	Synergies natural to the community
Individual creativity	Collective creativity
Market research (audience surveys)	Participatory research & evaluation
Fixed product	Process theatre
Star system	Community actors

---

[2] Walter Benjamin, *Understanding Brecht* (London & New York: Verso, 1998): 1–13; David Kerr & Stephen Chifunyise, "Popular Theatre in Zambia: Chikwakwa Reassessed," *Theatre International* 11–12 (1984): 75–76.

[3] David Kerr, *African Popular Theatre from Pre-Colonial Times to the Present Day* (London: James Currey, 1995): 172; PETA, *Mamugnaong Dula/Creative Dynamics* (Davao City: MCPCS, 1980).

Although this set of binaries has obvious elements of truth, there is much over-simplification designed to demonize media imperialism.

I would like to expand a little on the media categories, because I shall return to them later in this essay. One of the most powerful tools of multinational media companies is their deployment of huge resources to research market segmentation and changes in tastes. Another is the way they mobilize a variety of media platforms in order to support its product through the synergies of its various sections. Thus, Disney's ownership of a huge cinema production and distribution system (and much more) is supported by television stations, radio stations, sports shops, theme parks, cruise ships, recording studios, and record labels.[4] The films, records, radio programmes, brand T-shirts, and other products support each other, with particular appeal to the young. For cultural workers in Africa, it seems occasionally like a hopeless struggle against what PR gurus call 'total communication strategies', especially as Northern corporate media are astute at disguising the manipulative aspects of their own organization and practices.

Returning to my narrative, by the late 1980s the practical application of my anti-imperialist binary paradigm became more difficult once applied-theatre activists in Africa had to come to terms with issues of HIV/AIDS. My first realization of this came in 1987 when I attended a hastily called workshop for journalists, broadcasters, and popular communication workers, organized by the World Health Organisation in Blantyre, Malawi. At the workshop, many faith-based communicators refused point-blank to associate with any messages advocating the use of condoms, and some interpreted the virus as God's punishment for human sin. The debates between secular WHO facilitators and faith-based communicators seemed distressingly far from the struggles that had engaged me for the previous two decades.

My own crisis came as a result of not being able to fit issues of HIV/AIDS into my comfort-zone paradigm of cultural imperialism at war with defenders of local cultural democracy. In short, I craved for some entity to blame, but, short of accepting conspiracy theories about mad American scientists or of cursing some vengeful god, there was no-one to blame. Theatrically, that seemed to mean being forced into a space I had hitherto firmly resisted, that of pure instrumentalism.

---

[4] Benjamin M. Compaine & Douglas Gongery, *Who Owns the Media? Competition and Concentration in the Mass Media Industry* (Mahwah NJ & London: Lawrence Erlbaum Associates, 2000): 313.

The first HIV/AIDS play I helped to devise (shortly after the 1987 WHO workshop) was with a small, all-male group of drama students in Zomba, Malawi. We brainstormed various ideas until we settled on a loose plot-line. I had recently shown the students a video of Mbongeni Ngema's devised play *Asinamali*.[5] The students decided to take the idea of a prison frame within which inmates told the stories of how they were imprisoned, and adapt it to a TB ward in a Malawian public hospital, with the patients telling each other how they thought they were infected with HIV. For me, the play harboured problems, because, unlike *Asinamali*, the stories failed to accumulate the kind of energy that could convert pity into anger, since it was not clear where the anger could be directed. Another problem was that the students were very ignorant of many issues about HIV/AIDS. This was consistent with the characters they played, but led to the ethical dilemma that they might be recycling myths to the audiences. I tried to rectify this to some extent, but had constantly to consult with friends in the medical profession.

This last issue is one of many that I believe gave support to the rise of mediated drama as funding agencies' preferred methodology for educating African communities about HIV/AIDS. Many NGOs in the late 1980s and early 1990s realized that the participatory techniques of applied theatre gave rise to a danger of false information being recycled in communities. One solution to the problem was to train theatre workers in the fundamental medical facts about HIV/AIDS; this had a double pay-off, in that, in addition to acquiring medical information, such trained actors, facilitators, and playwrights tended to develop a strong commitment to issues concerning the virus.

However, another dynamic militated against such a process: the imperative of budgets, targets, and action-plan indicators. These factors encouraged many NGOs to invest in such media as radio or television drama, documentaries, and talk shows, which could reach greater numbers than live theatre, and, even more crucially, could be closely monitored to ensure that theatrical discourse conformed to medical accuracy.

This shift in emphasis coincided with other transitions taking place in the political economy of NGO management. The spread of corporate project-management methods in the private sector during the Reagan–Thatcher era of the 1980s began to influence communication-oriented NGOs. By 1990 market research, project proposals, strategic plans, log-frames, communica-

---

[5] Mbongeni Ngema, "Asinamali!" in *Woza Afrika! An Anthology of South African Plays*, ed. Duma Ndlhovu (New York: George Braziller, 1986): 177–224.

tion design, performance evaluation, and, most of all, monitoring and evaluation became the language which even the most anarchic and spontaneous artists had to learn in order to obtain funding. Very few drama activists were able to span the creative and managerial roles this shift in emphasis demanded. In the field of HIV/AIDS education, the holistic approach to health-oriented theatre that I had enjoyed in the 1970s and 1980s gave way to a system of task demarcations and restrictive practices, with creative artists having to slot their skills into a communication strategy worked out by communication specialists, sometimes far from the 'target' communities.

The theoretical gains which theatre activists had struggled to achieve in the 1980s came under threat. Where we had pushed for the participation of the community in problem identification, research, play-making, performance, monitoring, and evaluation, many NGOs began to insist on a disaggregation of these roles. In addition, the imperative to quantify HIV/AIDS messaging in the most cost-efficient ways tended to validate media such as radio drama and mobile video shows rather than live theatre.

I do not want to cast myself as a Luddite on this issue. I can see the usefulness of, for example, trying to build systematic monitoring and evaluation practices into drama campaigns, whether live or mediated. My problem is the tendency for some project management methods to disempower communities in order to ensure that they are guided in the direction of appropriate changes in behaviour.

But in order to avoid appearing like an intellectual Luddite, let me concentrate on a few mediated drama projects which, I feel, contain considerable empowering elements as well as troubling tendencies. In the process I hope to identify some of the strengths as well as weaknesses of media campaigns.

One of the most interesting projects in which I got involved in the late 1990s in Botswana was a video drama called *Bonang*, for which I served as an advisor. A youthful Francistown theatre group called Ghetto Artists, led by my former student Vuyisele Otukile, created the play in 1997 in conjunction with, and funded by, the AIDS/STD Unit of the Botswana Ministry of Health. The play was aimed at secondary schools and youth groups in order to encourage either abstinence or responsible sex.

Otukile was very familiar with Boalian techniques of audience participation from his theatre training and practice.[6] He decided to make the video

---

[6] Vuyisele Otukile, "Community Theatre for HIV/AIDS Social Treatment in Botswana" (MA thesis, University of Botswana, Gaborone, 2006).

version of the play interactive through use of a double screening. The first time the video was shown all the way through, without any intervention. Then the facilitators showed it a second time and stopped at various pre-planned key moments, when characters were faced with a choice. This allowed the facilitators to engage with the audience in discussion about the choices facing the characters. A facilitators' handbook that accompanied the video made suggestions on how to manage the question-and-answer sessions.

This technique allowed some of the advantages of participatory theatre to be captured, though others were lost. The modification to Ghetto Artists' script was particularly problematic, since each scene had to be vetted by a six-person committee of doctors, social workers, counsellors, and PHC nurses. As opposed to the enthusiastic, collective creativity I had become used to in community playmaking, the strong bureaucratic tendencies of this committee diluted the dramatic impact of some of the scenes.

Shortly after the *Bonang* project, Otukile became the director of a health-based NGO called the Youth Health Organisation (YOHO). The funding made available to him through such US funding agencies as AED[7] and BOTUSA[8] allowed YOHO to develop a variety of media in order to create a 'total-communication' impact. Thus, campaigns on such issues as voluntary counselling and testing were covered through participatory stage drama, dance-mime, radio drama, radio round-tables, posters, travelling events, and a website.

'Total-communication' campaigns have become a feature of media-based strategies in Southern Africa. Naturally, such large-scale organization requires an equally large organizational base and methodology. US funding and management systems have played a crucial role in shaping African communication about HIV. Johns Hopkins University has provided considerable leadership and funding in this field, with its communication concepts promulgated through the Drumbeat Communication Initiative Network website and Newsletter (Communication Initiative).

The jewel in the crown of the Johns Hopkins ideological empire is the Johannesburg-based Soul City Institute for Development and Health Communication, which is famous for its popular television drama series *Soul City*.

---

[7] Academy for Educational Development, a US NGO and funding agency based in Salt Lake City.

[8] "Botswana-USA" is another health-based NGO/funding agency (mostly channelling USAID funds) dealing with health issues.

With support from the British Government and other donors, the Institute also uses a variety of media, including radio, magazines, live events, pop concerts, a fashion company, and a website. In addition, the Soul City brand, with its administrative apparatus of research and evaluation, is exported through similar communication strategies to other countries in the region.

I would like to pay particular attention to a similar media-driven communication campaign in Botswana. The project, *Makgabaneng*, is principally a radio soap opera broadcast twice a week on Radio Botswana, and is also linked to Johns Hopkins University, though not directly to Soul City. One of my Media students, upon graduation, was employed as a scriptwriter for *Makgabaneng*, which allowed me fairly close contact with the organization. The soap opera has a well-drilled set of procedures and drama packaging, and is aimed at a clear market niche – teenagers and young adults. One of the remarkable features of *Makgabaneng* is the extreme youth of most of its workers, including trainers, producers, and particularly actors.

Some of the senior workers have been trained in the Johns Hopkins method, which seeks to link the aesthetics of the drama-creation process with medical or social research and theory. The ideology even has an uplifting militaristic name, MARCH (Modeling and Reinforcement to Combat HIV/AIDS). Cognitive communication theory is the bedrock on which the soap opera is built, in particular the five stages which an ignorant or recalcitrant character goes through while being convinced of the need for a change of behaviour.[9] The 'Stages of Change' are, in ascending order of self-awareness: Precontemplation, Contemplation, Preparation, Action, and Maintenance. Although someone may progress from one to another, he/she can also backslide, and, since it is a soap opera, often does.

The scriptwriters go through rigorous training in order to blend their creative skills with the socio-medical issues.[10] When the scriptwriters get together, they start with the medical and social messages, as well as the crucial psychological dilemmas or turning points which determine the direction a character will take. The messages (or "formative themes") are given labels (from A to

[9] Maungo Mooki, "Makgabaneng Re Wa Re Tsoga and Reinforcement Activities: An HIV/AIDS Behaviour Change Intervention in Botswana" (PowerPoint presentation for Media Studies Conference on Media Edutainment, University of Botswana, Gaborone, 2006): frame 13.

[10] Mooki, "Makgabaneng Re Wa Re Tsoga and Reinforcement Activities: An HIV/AIDS Behaviour Change Intervention in Botswana," frame 18.

F) and each episode is designed to provide exposure to some of these messages.[11] The whole process involves much committee work, monitoring, and design of tables for themes or character development.

As would be expected, the *Makgabaneng* researchers undertake thorough evaluation, which in its published form takes the shape of tables indicating the extent to which audience exposure to *Makgabaneng* has affected the various indices.[12]

My account of *Makgabaneng* so far may suggest a very manipulative unidirectional model of communication, where programmatic logic outweighs collective creativity. However, the designers of the campaign are aware of the need for constructive feedback, not only for the purpose of qualitative research but also to find alternative, interactive methods of reinforcing the messages. For this purpose, there are various other media, including a website, road shows (with popular musicians and dance groups), a board game (called "Pathways to Change"), a network of school clubs, management of a hot-line for emergency counselling, and a successful magazine (*Teen Mag*). The magazine encourages feedback about the radio drama through letters or interactive photo-novellas. In addition, the *Makgabaneng* institution has very close ties with other relevant NGOs (particularly Childline) in order that the counselling section can provide referral services.

Even though there are no institutional links with Soul City, I think it is easy to see the similarity in the use of total-communication techniques, the carefully planned research, the methodological aesthetics of story-creation, and the very thorough, statistical evaluation.

In my references to *Makgabaneng* and Soul City I am aware that my language is occasionally pejorative, in applying commercial phrases such as 'media empire', 'template', 'brand', 'packaging', and 'market niche'. Admittedly, I do find aspects of these communication campaigns rather disturbing because of their close similarity to corporate communication strategies, the evil empire I had demonized in the 1970s. I focus on three in particular:

1) NGOs target African communities through media convergence, synergies and other marketing techniques in a strategy similar to

[11] Mooki, "Makgabaneng Re Wa Re Tsoga and Reinforcement Activities," frame 15.

[12] Katina Pappas–DeLuca, Todd Koppenhaver and the Makgabaneng Listenership Survey Group, 2005, *Makgabaneng Radio Serial Drama Listenership Survey Report, Botswana* (Research Report, Republic of Botswana and BOTUSA, Gaborone, 2005).

multinational corporations such as Disney, Times Warner, and News Corp.

2) Soul City has an 'empire' of satellite organizations in the peripheries of South Africa; the institutional convergencies and financial complexity of these relationships is disturbingly similar to US, European or East Asian media centres controlling communication franchises in the peripheries of global private sector networks.
3) The communication methodologies are instigated by Northern NGO 'think-tanks', which, through the transfer of methodology, are then applied to African communities, to the possible detriment of local aesthetic autonomy.

With all three of these concerns I have an ambiguous attitude. Is it a question of NGO communicators smartly assuming a policy of 'If you can't beat them join them'? Or are the strategies a sign of multinational corporations infiltrating African development institutions in order to transfer corporate communication methods?

Whatever my instinct to recoil, I have become cautious about attempting to castigate *Makgabaneng* and Soul City. At a basic level, if these communication strategies actually work and save lives it is difficult to criticize them. Another, more culture-based reason is that these practices have now become almost wholly localized – thus, what may have started as a neo-colonial import is well on the way to becoming as much a part of local hybrid culture as *kwaito*, football, or Nigerian video dramas. A further argument is that mediated drama, music, comics, and dance have, whether professors like it or not, become highly popular, particularly among the young, and it makes sense to mobilize the power of such communication tools even if this appears to undermine African indigenous culture.

The whole argument about authenticity becomes particularly ambiguous when we look at new media. It is clear that in the twenty-first century the romanticized notion of local African communities sitting around fires preserving indigenous culture, while still viable, has been transformed by modernization. In some ways, such societies are becoming articulated with other types of virtual community, particularly cell-phone networks, but also social networking sites and chat rooms. Just as the multinational corporations have been quick to latch onto the potential of e-commerce, so local NGOs like Soul City and Makgabaneng have, as part of their total communication strategy, used their websites to provide discussion groups and blogs.

I'd like to quote from a specific blog on the Soul City satellite project *One Love*, which is a communication campaign about multi-concurrent partnerships. The comments are a tiny, unedited sample of responses to issues raised in the Malawian *One Love* blog about issues concerning multi-concurrent partners (MCPs).

> Bundule's Response, Posted August 13, 2009 at 2:59 pm | Permalink
> whats funny is when its the spare wheel the sky is the limit all position are tried to the maximum koma kunyumba nde missionary always. hehehe well no much to comment but alos ladies need to open up koz they pretend not to know anything at the begining of the relatonship when they re the masters in bed, so one gets suprised to learnt that the same person who didnt know a thing about sex overnight she is the master of them all. how come ladies reply on this. MCP will always be there wherther your satisfied at home or not, because MCP's dont come because of sex only but other issues as well like time management by ladies, too much noise in the house, nagging, not respecting other pples phones, and not spoiling the man enough, u let the man wonder around and take a cold bath when ur busy watching tv, thats when spare tyres are needed. to feel the gap left by the flat tyre at home.
>
> Grace's Response Posted August 14, 2009 at 1:27 pm | Permalink
> Bundule you realy have a way with words. I couldn't help but smile when I was reading through your comment. The issue of MCP is very complex. As you pointed out some poeple will start MCP not because of sexual dissatisfaction...NO! But because of other factors such as a nagging spouse etc. However I think sexual dissatsfaction is one of the most important factor that drives both men and women into MCP. Wholistically speaking though i think we should be aiming at having solid relationships in every aspect of the word. A relationship that is sexually, emotionally, socially and spiritually satisfying. As a relationship we should be able to communicate all issues whether its sex, or something as simple as watching movies. we should be able to address our issues amicably without having to nag all the time. as I said this is a complex issue but it starts with us taking one step in making that relationship work. Eeee lets pump up the flat tyres so that we don't resolve to use the spare one.[13]

---

[13] One Love Blog "Soul City" (30 October 2009), www.onelovesouthernafrica org /index.php/Malawians-say-men-prefer-women-who-are-skilled-in-bed (accessed 30 October 2009).

What I find interesting about the blog is that the discourse sounds utterly Malawian, with its code-switching between English and Chichewa, and its good-humoured bantering between male and female 'roles'. The blog discussion refers to realities of Malawian sexual culture but within a frame that accepts the rapid changes taking place. An interaction of this nature would be almost unimaginable in some village assemblies in Malawi, though it is imaginable in others. The point is that the virtual community of the blog, where the participants may not even be physically in Malawi, raises productive (but also sometimes dangerous) possibilities for a virtual participatory audience to push discussions about sexuality into taboo areas. At the same time, many participants in the debate are presumably also interacting with 'real' Malawian communities, so that both the African and non-African sources of hybridity are kept in a state of continuous interaction. It is possible to imagine that the relatively democratic space of blogs, tweets, and chat rooms can provide a forum which reconstitutes aspects of the free-flowing Freirian forum that theatre practitioners valorized in the 1970s and 1980s.

My current attitude, therefore, about use of media in HIV/AIDS communication is to accept it as inevitable, recognizing its power to influence people but making a few recommendations to ensure that the most instrumental aspects of mediated communication do not destroy the aesthetic riches and indigenous African creativity which theatre practitioners have drawn upon and encouraged over the years.

1) It is very important for African thinkers and communicators to develop their own theories of communication, particularly in the complex relationships between messages, facilitation, media aesthetics, and funders. This is not to say that such communicators need to jettison all theories which have been developed by Northern 'think tanks', since many of those ideas originated or were developed in Africa. But it is necessary for African communication on HIV/AIDS issues to build ownership of their core theories by constantly testing them with realities on the ground.
2) One important aspect of such theorizing would be to find ways of preventing the reification of HIV/AIDS issues. At present, many dramas, whether live or mediated, place excessive emphasis on instrumental solutions (such as fidelity, condoms, abstinence or male circumcision) without placing such solutions in the complex fabric of African social life. The issues need to be interwoven with a perspective that foregrounds global and micro-economic inequalities,

social othering, and cultural insecurities. For example, we need to recognize the usefulness of mainstreaming HIV/AIDS by creating broad-based dramas in which HIV/AIDS is only one of many thematic strands.

3) Dialogue is needed between African live-theatre workers and those in media communication. This would entail accepting the economies of scale and the glamour provided by media communication while building synergies with the participatory, adaptable qualities of face-to-face communication. It also means strategizing around an afrocentric version of 'total communication' where innovative methods of interactive media practice can provide productive support for 'oramedia'.
4) Particular attention needs to be paid to new media such as blogs, Twitter, social networking sites, listserves, and chat-rooms in order to research the positive and negative aspects of emergent, digital global communications. This has to be achieved through ways which do not widen the 'digital gap' but which instead can articulate productively with 'real communities' on the ground.

I realize that these recommendations only begin to address in a small way the complexity of communication issues about HIV/AIDS, and I am simply putting some items on a long pedagogical agenda rather than solving problems. The journey that has led me to this point has taken me away from the over-simplistic binaries that motivated me in the 1970s. But the increased self-doubts, confusions, and soul-searching that I now face in the twenty-first century have not blunted my conviction that medical problems necessarily relate to broader aspects of global injustice and struggle. I believe that addressing this tangle of disguised links and articulations requires even more commitment than when the enemy seemed easy to identify.

WORKS CITED

Benjamin, Walter. *Understanding Brecht* (London & New York: Verso, 1998).

Compaine, Benjamin M., & Douglas Gongery. *Who Owns the Media? Competition and Concentration in the Mass Media Industry* (Mahwah NJ & London: Lawrence Erlbaum Associates, 2000).

Kerr, David. *African Popular Theatre from Pre-Colonial Times to the Present Day* (London: James Currey,1995).

——. *Dance, Media Entertainment & Popular Theatre in South East Africa* (Bayreuth African Studies 43; Bayreuth: Eckhard Breitinger, 1996).

——, & Stephen Chifunyise. "Popular Theatre in Zambia: Chikwakwa Reassessed," *Theatre International* 11–12 (1984): 54–80.

Magalasi, Mufunanji. "Stage Drama in Independent Malawi: 1980 to 2002" (doctoral dissertation, University of Malawi, Zomba, 2006).

Mooki, Maungo. "Makgabaneng Re Wa Re Tsoga and Reinforcement Activities: An HIV/AIDS Behaviour Change Intervention in Botswana" (PowerPoint presentation, for Media Studies Conference on Media Edutainment, University of Botswana, Gaborone, 2006).

Ngema, Mbongeni. "Asinamali!" in *Woza Afrika! An Anthology of South African Plays*, ed. Duma Ndlhovu (New York: George Braziller, 1986): 177–24.

Otukile, Vuyisele. "Community Theatre for HIV/AIDS Social Treatment in Botswana" (MA thesis, University of Botswana, Gaborone, 2006).

Pappas–DeLuca, Katina, Todd Koppenhaver and the Makgabaneng Listenership Survey Group. *Makgabaneng Radio Serial Drama Listenership Survey Report, Botswana* (Research Report, Republic of Botswana and BOTUSA, Gaborone, 2005).

PETA. *Mamugnaong Dula/Creative Dynamics* (Davao City: MCPCS, 1980).

Website References

The Communication Initiative Network, www.communit.com (accessed 11 October 2009).

Johns Hopkins University Project South Africa, http//broadcasthivafrica/org/docs/summary_of_USAID-Hopkins_Study.pdf (accessed 30 October 2009).

One Love Blog. *Soul City*, www.onelovesouthernafrica.org/index.php/Malawians-say-men-prefer-women-who-are-skilled-in-bed (accessed 30 October 2009).

Soul City. www.soulcity.org.za (accessed 30 October 2009).

YOHO. www.communit.com/en/node/121030 (accessed 30 October 2009).

⌘

Innovations in Research Approaches

EMELDA NGUFOR SAMBA

Appreciative Inquiry

An Alternative Approach to Applied Theatre

APPLIED THEATRE, be it community theatre or theatre for development, has for many years been acclaimed as one of the most successful approaches to reaching out to disadvantaged rural and urban communities. This success has been enhanced by the participatory nature of applied theatre, especially in situations where the inside-out and bottom-top methods have been given prominence. In Africa, and other developing countries, applied theatre is considered as an appropriate medium to reach out to communities, both urban and rural, that are challenged by social, cultural, and economic issues. This approach has been particularly successful in cases where communities have been deeply implicated, from the conception to the implementation stages of community projects. Through this medium, communities have had the chance to become aware of their very essence through reflection, dialogue, story-creation, and performance. So far, the core of the African theatre for development approach has been the problem-posing and problem-solving rooted in the Freirean pedagogy of the oppressed.

As a practitioner in the field, I have registered relative success with communities faced with difficult situations in the areas of politics, health, culture, and economics. Through the problem-posing method, communities have come to a recognition of their limited situations and the possibilities available to overcome them. Inspiring conversations have taken place, lived experiences narrated, alternative ways of resolving problems suggested, with all these culminating in improvised performances; performances acclaimed for their verisimilitude in identifying and analysing community problems.

What has also been noticed during theatre for development workshops is the tendency to blame oneself and others for the relative lack of success in certain aspects of community life. Parents have tended to blame children's poor performances on the indiscipline in schools, and teachers have blamed this same relative lack of success on inappropriate home training. In other cases, villagers have blamed the absence of community development on the poor leadership qualities of the village chiefs, whereas the local chiefs have at the same time considered the villagers rebellious and uncooperative. Disabled people, for their part, have poured out their frustration, branding the non-physically challenged, including institutions, as insensitive to their problems.[1] This, they have argued, has manifested itself in the inaccessibility of public buildings and negative discrimination by employers.

Workshops with HIV/AIDS-infected persons have also had their stories of blame–blame discussions. Much time has been spent answering questions and justifying certain decisions and actions by government officials, HIV/AIDS-infected and affected persons, and those who stigmatize them. Facilitators have often been hooked up with communities in the process of identifying problems, prioritizing them, and analysing them, all this in a bid to arrive at a reconciliatory stance. Seemingly satisfactory solutions have been offered and facilitators have often gone home with the conviction that they have brought the community to a certain level of consciousness.

Talking against problem-posing education, the International Institute for Sustainable Development explicates this better when it states that, generally, development agencies

> generate volumes of data that provide great detail on the origins and consequences of local needs and resource constraints. Interventions to address the problems are then developed, usually by consulting with the local community. But at the end of such an approach local people, not surprisingly, often view their community as a place full of problems and needs, most of which require the help of outsiders to overcome. By creating and reinforcing this identity through ongoing exercises during the project cycle, these approaches could have a disempowering effect that contributes to the development workers being viewed as the agents of change in the community, rather than the community members themselves. This viewpoint establishes and en-

---

[1] Emelda Ngufor Samba, "Enabling the Disabled through Theatre," *Leeds African Studies Bulletin* 67 (March 2005): 46–57.

> trenches a sense of dependency in the community that the agency must then work to overcome.[2]

The above passage highlights some of the challenges that resource persons and facilitators of applied theatre have to deal with every so often. So far, some of the main challenges with applied theatre are how facilitators and resource persons can enable communities to have more life-giving conversations. How can they approach applied theatre in a way that is more empowering and fulfilling to both facilitators and communities? How to ask questions that would lead communities to focus on their strengths, their potentials, and what is working in their communities in a way that gives them the feeling that they, not the facilitators, are the agents of change? My involvement as a facilitator in the British Council InterAction Leadership Programme[3] put me in touch with Appreciative Inquiry, which could provide some answers to these concerns.

Appreciative Inquiry is a socio-constructivist theory developed by David Cooperrider and Diana Whitney.[4] They see it as a positive revolution for change that focuses on what is working to bring about changes in living systems. It is the

> study and exploration of what gives life to human systems when they function at their best. It is based on the assumption that every living system has a hidden and underutilized core of strength – its positive core – which when revealed and tapped, provides a sustainable source of positive energy for both personal and organizational transformation.[5]

In the appreciative core, valuing, prizing, esteeming, and honouring are synonymous with 'appreciate', while discovery, search, systematic explora-

---

[2] International Institute for Development, *Appreciative Inquiry and Community Development* (2000).

[3] The InterAction Leadership Programme, until it came to an end in 2008, was considered one of the British Council's most prestigious programmes on leadership. Developed by Africans, the programme forged the way forward for revolutionary leadership and had as its base, Appreciative Inquiry.

[4] David Cooperrider & Diane Whitney, *A Positive Revolution to Change: Appreciative Inquiry* (San Francisco: Berrett–Koehler, 2005).

[5] James D. Ludema, Bernard J. Mohr & Diane Whitney, *Appreciative Inquiry Summit: A Practitioner's Guide for Leading Large Group Change* (San Francisco: Berret–Koehler, 2000): 9.

tion, and study are synonymous with 'inquiry'. Putting these synonyms together, I venture to define Appreciative Inquiry as a systematic exploration and study of a community, organization, and situation in a way that lends it value, esteem, and honour. If we take this as our working definition, then our conversations in applied theatre, be this community theatre or theatre for development, would move away from identifying and analysing community problems towards identifying, analysing, valuing, and honouring communities' strengths and successes that have enhanced self-esteem and honour. The stories told in improvised performances would therefore be stories that speak to the strengths and potentials of the communities; stories of past successes and of how the collective effort of the community contributed to this success.

Appreciative Inquiry is both a theory and a practice, and at its core are the 4-D Cycle and its eight key assumptions. The purpose of this essay is to explore the potential benefits of experimenting with Appreciative Inquiry as an alternative approach to the problem-posing and problem-solving approach that has so far been at the service of applied theatre. Considering that applied theatre is known for the flexibility of its methodology, the essay further seeks to challenge theatre practitioners to consider experimenting with this alternative in their interaction with communities challenged by difficult situations. For better comprehension, this essay will review two of the key concepts in Appreciative Inquiry: its eight assumptions, and the 4-D Cycle.

The Eight Assumptions of Appreciative Inquiry

Appreciative Inquiry holds that at every given point in our lives we make numerous assumptions about people and situations. These assumptions, it argues, guide our modes of behaviour. If this is so, then we must be watchful of the kinds of assumptions we entertain about organizations, communities, individuals, and situations. Theatre practitioners working with communities often hold views about the people, the issues at stake, and the institutions. Being much more critical of the assumptions they hold of situations before, during, and after their field experiences inevitably guides them as they facilitate conversations and improvise plays with communities. Appreciative Inquiry highlights eight key assumptions that, it is believed, would, if held, enable people to work with the best of themselves and others in any given situation. In this section, I will attempt to explain how these key assumptions can be of use to applied-theatre practitioners.

1. In every organization, situation or individual, something works.

This assumption is the key to the appreciative core. Getting into every situation knowing that something works gives people opportunities to seek the strength and successes of others. Theatre-for-development practitioners who approach a community adhering to this assumption would tend to first seek what is working in that community and the factors contributing to the community's achievements. By asking workshop participants to identify and analyse their community or organization's strength rather than their problems, facilitators might be giving them a lifetime opportunity to seek the good in themselves and other people. This becomes crucial especially in workshops with participants who feel marginalized and rejected and have lost self esteem. Disabled people, HIV/AIDS-infected persons, battered women, prisoners, rape victims. and even displaced communities who have lost or are in the process of losing self-esteem might find this approach enabling and empowering. HIV/AIDS-infected persons, for instance, would be acknowledging their potentials rather than lamenting their stigmatization. They might want to focus on the few sympathetic people rather than on those who act as a constant reminder of their HIV/AIDS status. Acknowledging that something works in the system despite all else could act as a driving force to motivate self and others in similar or worse conditions. Whitney and Cooperrider argue that, when one links the positive core to any agenda for change, changes never thought possible are suddenly and democratically mobilized.

2. What we focus on becomes our reality.

Deciding what we want for ourselves and our community is the first step towards achieving it. Given the limited time that is often allocated for real interaction in applied-theatre projects, it becomes useful for facilitators to focus communities' attention on their dreams and help them plan to achieve these dreams. Allocating more time for people to revisit community achievements and to review the strategies employed to arrive at those achievements, and focusing on what they want to achieve rather than on their problems could produce more sustainable and beneficial outcomes.

3. People move in the directions to which they are questioned.

The questions people ask themselves, organizations, and individuals often lead them to particular actions and decisions. Whereas 'how?' and 'what would be different?' questions create opportunities for creativity and put both questioner and the questioned in a safe container to carry out life-giving conversations, 'why?' questions, by contrast, put the person interrogated in a defensive mode and tend to stifle creativity. Appreciative Inquiry focuses on affirmatively disruptive questions, those questions that completely change one's way of perceiving situations. Affirmatively disruptive questions would make workshop participants pause for a while to reflect on their day-to-day routines and the benefits that would accrue if their activities and strengths were better streamlined towards community mobilization and empowerment. In a conflict situation, for instance, a question like 'How would the community benefit when it has resolved this issue?' is likely to make members of the community see themselves as people capable of achieving remarkable success. Visualizing the benefits that come when a solution is arrived at acts as a motivating force for constructing dialogue.

4. The language we use creates our reality.

Individuals have the choice to use the language of the creator or the language of the judge or destroyer. The language of the creator creates opportunities for people in difficult situations to explore new grounds and overcome the limits of situations. Such a language speaks to self-esteem and is empowering. Telling people they are capable and that their successes depend on them opens up opportunities for new thinking and positive action. Conversely, using judgmental language or language that diminishes self-respect is oppressive. Facilitators therefore have the challenge of regulating the language used by community members, especially in conflict situations.

5. Reality is created in the moment and there are multiple realities.

Keeping in mind that people have different backgrounds and that different experiences guide people's interpretation of events puts facilitators in a mode to understand and accommodate people better. Additionally, acknowledging that reality is created in the moment compels one to seek an understanding of what makes people 'tick' at every given time. Time, content, and the internal become recognized as elements that condition people's reactions and behaviour at any given time. Holding onto this assumption would inevitably urge facilitators to carry out more profound research into the situation they have to intervene in. This will also enable them to have a more open mind to appreciate the different points of view of the various stakeholders.

6. We should value the magic of difference.

What makes the rainbow magical are the different colours that constitute it. Every human system is made up of people of different ages, sex, educational background, and socio-political leanings. Facilitators who enter a project with this in mind and with the preparedness to include all these different groups are more likely to get the best out of the community. Workshops that are more inclusive of different categories of people are likely to benefit from diverse experiences and are subsequently more rewarding.

7/8 People move into the future with parts of the past/ When we move into the future, we should carry the best of our past with us.

In her book *And Then You Act*, Anne Bogart draws attention to Antjie Krog's description of a poet as that person who "remembers where the water holes are."[6] Memory, for an artist, is a great requirement, and Appreciative Inquiry recommends that we move forward with the best of what we can remember. Considering that past successes and achievements kindle aspirations towards future greater achievements, it becomes the responsibility of theatre practitioners, who are the catalysts of community mobilization, to focus communities' attention on those aspects of their history that brought them value, honour, and glory. The artist might remember where all the water holes are, but it rests on him to decide whether to lead the people to all the holes or take them to those water holes that produce clean, fresh water; holes that give life.

The Appreciative Cycle or the 4-D Cycle

Cooperrider and Whitney's appreciative cycle is made up of four stages: Discovery, which is about appreciating and valuing that which is; the Dream stage, which engages communities in envisioning what might be; Design, which entails co-constructing the future; and Destiny, which entails learning, empowering, and improvising to sustain the future. Augusto Boal's image theatre is closely linked to this model, although his transformation model has three images; the actual, the ideal, and the transitional.[7] Boal's actual image

---

[6] Anne Bogart, *And Then You Act: Making Art in an Unpredictable World* (New York: Routledge, 2007): 2.

[7] Augusto Boal, *Theatre of the Oppressed*, tr. Charles A. McBride, María–Odilia Leal McBride & Emily Fryer (*Teatro do oprimido e outras poéticas políticas*, 1975; London: Pluto, 1979): 135.

could be likened to the discovery phase of Appreciative Inquiry. However, while the latter focuses on appreciating and valuing what makes a living system alive, Boal guides communities towards unveiling the problems that exist in the community in a bid to solve them. This comes across strongly in the subject-matter of the plays presented by the Arena Theatre: "bribery in provincial soccer games, strikes against capitalists, adultery in a small village, subhuman living conditions of railway employees, bandits [...] in the Northeast."[8]

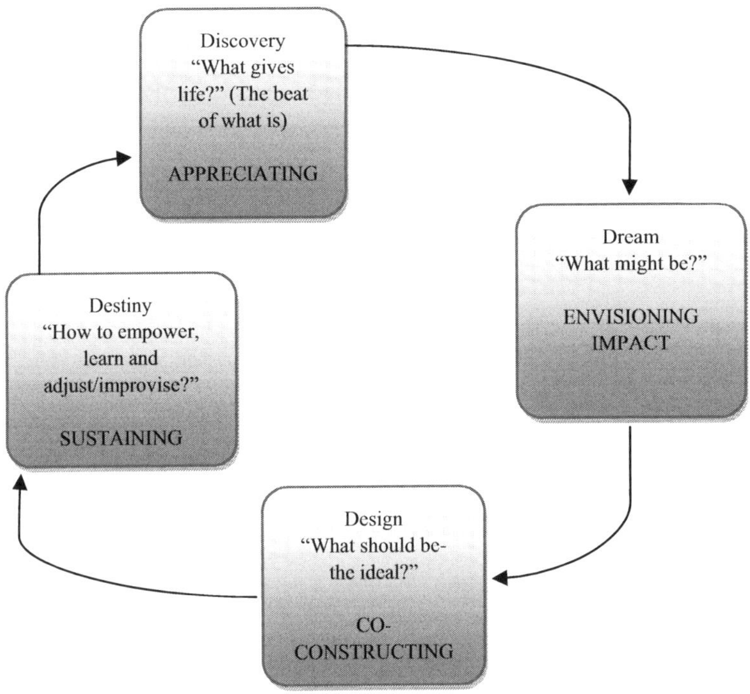

Figure 1: The four Ds of Cooperrider and Whitney[9]

[8] Boal, *Theatre of the Oppressed*, 163.

[9] The chart is copied from the International Institute for Sustainable Development, "Appreciative Inquiry and Community Development" (2000), http://www.iisd.org/ai (accessed 14 October 2009).

He says:

> When finally an image is arrived at that is the most acceptable to all, then the spectator sculptor is asked to show the way the given theme should be; that is in the first grouping, the *actual image* is shown, the second, the *ideal image*. Finally, he is asked to show a transitional *image*, to show how it would be possible to pass from one reality to the other. In other words, how to carry out the change, the transformation, the revolution, or what ever term one wishes to use.[10]

Likewise, Boal's ideal image can be likened to the dream stage of Appreciative Inquiry, for, in both cases, communities project into the future to visualize a system in a near-perfect state. The transitional and design phases give communities a chance to co-construct: i.e. to come up with plans that could produce the desired transformation. Appreciative Inquiry, however, offers resource persons something additional, a chance to begin again, and this at the Destiny stage. Being dynamic, living systems are in constant flux, in a search for the best in man and the environment. This accounts for the persistent endeavour to improve on that which is.

DISCOVERY: The choice of the community for most theatre-for-development projects has often been determined by the depth of that community's problems. Inasmuch as this factor is fundamental – otherwise why go to that community? – Appreciative Inquiry proposes a focus on the community's discovering its strengths and potentials. It challenges resource persons to see a community as a mystery to be discovered rather than as a problem to be solved. So far, the reverse has been the case. In one of Boal's experiments, the spectator is asked to "express his views on a certain theme of common interest [...] or it can be a local problem such as the lack of water."[11] Describing one of the images a spectator presented, Boal writes that it was "a terrible, pessimistic, defeatist image, but also a true reflection of something that had actually taken place."[12] Hansel Ndumbe Eyoh also shows his dedication to the problem-posing approach when, in describing the Kumba Workshop, he states:

---

[10] Boal, *Theatre of the Oppressed,* 135.

[11] *Theatre of the Oppressed,* 135.

[12] *Theatre of the Oppressed*, 136.

> Before the session rose, it was suggested that the students, without the assistance of the resource persons, prepare some improvisations based on the problems they have encountered in the field.[13]

In yet another review of a theatre-for-development project, Zakes Mda reiterates the problem-posing and the problem-solving approach that is recurrent in TfD projects:

> Using these structures, we have created plays that have involved the community members in naming their problems, and in mapping out a definite course of action to solve the problems.[14]

David Kerr also mentions a theatre workshop in Mulangali where "researchers created an improvised play on [...] health problems."[15] Then the emphasis was also the identification, analysis, and resolution of the problems: "The idea of all the plays was to draw the audience into a dialogue about the health problems raised by the drama."[16] I have done likewise in many of my field experiences with children, adults, and youths, where I mostly began by asking the workshop participants to identify, analyse, and prioritize their problems.

The above examples all confirm the assertion that the problem-posing and problem-solving approach to community mobilization has long been at the service of applied-theatre practitioners. Most HIV/AIDS people already live a life of frustration, dejection, and regret, and the last thing they want to be reminded of is their state of helplessness. Conversations around how well they have fared this far, their recent and previous achievements in spite of their state of health, how they have been able to give life to others in similar situations through counselling, the strength they bring to their families by just being there – all this is at the centre of the appreciative core. It would bring to their awareness the values they have and the contributions they can make to an HIV/AIDS-free and/or accommodating society.

The choice of a project topic immediately creates the reality of the workshop discussion. Cooperrider and Whitney strongly recommend affirmative

---

[13] Hansel Ndumbe Eyoh, *Hammocks to Bridges* (Yaoundé: Bet, 1984): 49.

[14] Zakes Mda, "Another Theatre of the Absurd," in *Theatre and Performance in Africa*, ed. Eckhard Breitinger (Bayreuth African Studies 31; Bayreuth: Eckhard Breitinger, 1994): 106.

[15] David Kerr, Dance, Media Entertainment and Popular Theatre in South East Africa (Bayreuth African Studies 43; Bayreuth: Eckhard Breitinger, 1998): 235.

[16] Kerr, *Dance, Media Entertainment and Popular Theatre in South East Africa*, 235.

topics that evoke accomplishment and success. I have often fallen into fallacy of improvising plays and giving them such titles as 'The Rejected' and 'Deadlock'. Communities become more empowered when, in the initial stages of a workshop, they are led to talk about the strengths, potentials, and achievements they are proud of rather than their failures.

Such strengths and potentials could be community mobilization for common projects, past peaceful negotiations with neighbouring communities in conflict situations, and leadership skills of the local chiefs. During this phase, too, communities might come to realize what they would have done differently to have produced more sustainable outcomes. These would emerge from stories and personal lived experiences in the communities. Stories linked to the positive core are empowering both to the storyteller and to the listener. The assumption that the language we use creates our realities and reality is created in the moment becomes functional at this stage of self-discovery.

DREAM: The second stage in the 4-D Cycle is the Dream stage, where communities and /or organizations are guided to envision what might be. Having discovered what level they are at in their socio-political and economic development – what Augusto Boal calls the Actual Image – communities are led to dream of what might be (what Boal terms the Ideal Image: i.e. the image of the society they would want to create for themselves, given the human and material resources at their disposal). It becomes absolutely necessary that the dream come from the community, for they and they alone can bring this dream to fruition. Physically challenged persons, for instance, can dream of integration in a society where institutions have been put in place to facilitate their mobility, a society with special-needs schools and one with an awareness of the challenges they face.

DESIGN: In the design stage, community members or workshop participants co-construct, planning together how to accomplish their dreams, identifying the human and material resources required, and deciding on the timeframe needed to accomplish them. This is what Augusto Boal terms the Transitional Image. Exploring the magic of difference – tapping the intellectual, physical, and material resources of the various sub-groups in a community – is beneficial as the facilitator guides the community to map out a plan of action for transformational change. By valuing the views of every workshop participant, the facilitator enhances a sense of responsibility and ownership of the transformation process within the community, and, when it is time for implementation, the collective strength generated during the Dream and Design stages reverberates in the community for its collective empowerment.

DESTINY: Destiny comes after days, weeks or years of hard work when communities would have experimented with their plans of action. At this stage, they want to find out what they have achieved so far. They want to revisit the techniques used. They want to evaluate how individual and collective commitment contributed to their collective success. It could be a group of women seeking to affirm their rights as human beings in a community. It could be youths mapping out a route for more tolerance towards HIV/AIDS-infected persons. It could be a village seeking better guidance from its leaders. What is important at this stage is that they have had some valued achievement that is empowering and from which they can build future plans. What is also important is that, within the positive core, they can identify areas for adjustment, areas that can be improved upon. We might term this the follow-up stage, in which participants return to the field to evaluate the work done and to map out a way forward. The question is: having gone this far, having achieved our dreams, what next? What is the best of what we have achieved? What could we have done differently? This leads the community to the beginning of the cycle: the Dream stage.

Conclusion: Appreciative Inquiry and Applied Theatre

I was on the third theatre-for-development project with inmates of the Centre for the Rehabilitation of the Disabled in a Etoug-Egbe, Yaounde, Cameroon. In the first project, we improvised a play which we entitled 'The Rejected'. The second play was entitled 'The Rejected II',[17] and the third 'Deadlock'. In all of these workshops, we had galvanized so much energy discussing the plight of the disabled. We had listened to their stories, stories of disillusionment, hatred, and bitterness towards family relations who had abandoned them when they needed them most. The inmates had also poured out their frustration with the government, which, they believed, was doing very little to integrate them into Cameroonian society. Each session had been heavy for us all, both resource persons and participants. We had tried to keep a straight face, not to show the pain we were feeling deep inside because of the dreary stories we were listening to. We persisted, creating plays around these problems, and of course had a good audience, to whom we transferred our bitterness. On this third project, during one of the final rehearsal sessions, one of the participants, a high-school student, addressing me as "Auntie," as the

[17] Emelda Ngufor Samba, "Enabling the Disabled through Theatre," 46–47.

children fondly called me, said: "I don't want to play the part of a disabled person anymore." "What part would you like to play?" I asked him. "The part of a medical doctor, a lawyer, anything but the part of a disabled person."

This experience came to me as an eye-opener. It became clear to me that there was something that I as a theatre-for-development facilitator could be doing differently. The play titles we had collectively chosen, 'The Rejected' and 'Deadlock', had done nothing but remind an already disillusioned community of their disadvantaged situation. The statement stayed with me for a long time as I asked myself whether other alternative approaches were available to reach out to people within limited situations in a way that makes them believe more in themselves.

Application of the appreciative frame in applied theatre would begin with an Affirmative Topic Choice. Cooperrider and Whitney, in their effort to assist an organization that has come up with a project proposal on the 'problem' of sexual harassment, asked the question: "What is it that you want to learn about and achieve with this whole intervention, and by when?" After some prompting, they got a satisfactory affirmative topic: "What we really want to see is the development of the new century organization – a model of high quality cross-gender relationships in the work place!"[18] What this project is modelling is the shift from focusing on the problems to focusing on the desired result. It is about moving away from dialogue that underscores the sufferings of people to dialogue that gives life, dialogue that empowers. The wording of a project topic or play title inevitably conditions how participants approach the entire project. For example, project topics like 'The negative effects of widowhood rights' and 'sexual harassment in the work place' already create a feeling of bias in the minds of those who consider themselves victims or guilty. In essence, applying the affirmative core in applied theatre would mean facilitating dialogue on what the community wants to achieve from the entire intervention. It would, as I mentioned earlier, mean seeing the community as a mystery to be discovered, not as a problem to be solved. It would entail creating plays that exhibit the appreciative mood – moving from discovery, through dream and design, and, finally, to destiny. Based on the play context, spec-actors would unconsciously join the appreciative mode during the post-performance discussions in order to forge ahead.

---

[18] Cooperrider & Whitney, *A Positive Revolution to Change*, 5.

WORKS CITED

Boal, Augusto. *Theatre of the Oppressed*, tr. Charles A. McBride, María–Odilia Leal McBride & Emily Fryer (*Teatro do oprimido e outras poéticas políticas*, 1975; London: Pluto, 1979).

Bogart, Anne. *And Then You Act: Making Art in an Unpredictable World* (New York: Routledge, 2007).

Cooperrider, David L., & Diana Whitney. *A Positive Revolution to Change: Appreciative Inquiry* (San Francisco: Berrett–Koehler, 2005).

International Institute for Development. *Appreciative Inquiry and Community Development* (2000).

Kerr, David. *Dance, Media Entertainment and Popular Theatre in South East Africa* (Bayreuth: Bayreuth African Studies 43, 1998).

Ludema, James D. et al. *Appreciative Inquiry Summit: A Practitioner's Guide for Leading Large Group Change* (San Francisco: Berret–Koehler, 2009).

Mda, Zakes. "Another Theatre of the Absurd," in *Theatre and Performance in Africa*, ed. Eckhard Breitinger (Bayreuth: Bayreuth African Studies 31, 1994): 105–22.

Samba, Emelda Ngufor. "Enabling the Disabled through Theatre," *Leeds African Studies Bulletin* 67 (March 2005): 46–57.

⌘

GORDON BILBROUGH

After the Curtain – Reframed

Using Action Research to Reflect, Monitor, and Evaluate the Applied-Theatre Experience

THIS ESSAY EXAMINES arepp:Theatre for Life's use of action research as a framework for attempting to understand, capture, monitor, and evaluate the impact of its applied-theatre work and its value. The arepp:Theatre for Life Trust is an applied-theatre organization which has been operating nationally in South Africa since 1987. Using dramatic theatre presentations, arepp:Theatre for Life creates productions which travel to schools nation-wide, providing complementary social life-skills education to school-going learners for the promotion and development of self-efficacy and resilience in relation to sexuality and the attendant attitudes, behaviours, values, and views that are inherent therein.

Using a rights-based approach and presented in the real-life context of the audience, the productions have two aspects: the performance of a roughly thirty-minute play, and a subsequent thirty-minute facilitated discussion with the audience. The productions are specifically designed to be performed as a life-orientation lesson in the schools' daily schedule and to complement and support the outcomes of the national life-orientation curriculum and the strategic plan for HIV and AIDS.

Using an action L-learning approach, research, monitoring, and evaluation are embedded in every level of the intervention. In addition, nine external evaluations of the project have been completed to date. These all demonstrate clear evidence that the approach encourages and promotes openness, plain speaking, and debate; shows a positive improvement in such areas as understanding about HIV/AIDS information, gender equality, views on relationships, choice-making skills, tolerance of making mistakes, and self-esteem; and that the arepp:Theatre for Life interventions do increase a sense of self-efficacy with regard to sexuality in the audiences.[1]

Action research, participant action research, or action learning, as it is more recently being termed in development circles, is inquiry or research in the context of focused efforts to improve the quality of an organization and its performance. It is typically designed and conducted by practitioners who analyse the data to improve their own practice.[2] Action research involves cycles of planning, acting, data-collecting, and reflection on the part of the participants in the activity. The cycles are prompted by practical problems, issues, or questions that arise from the experience, the praxis, and which possibly indicate that the practice may need to change or adapt to achieve its desired outcomes.[3] Action research has the specific goal of improving the performance quality of the community or the area of concern, with the goal of

---

[1] Gordon Bilbrough, "After the Curtain: Designing an Impact Monitoring and Evaluation System for an Edutainment Theatre Intervention" (unpublished report, arepp:Theatre for Life: Cape Town, 2004); Gordon Bilbrough, "What Difference Does It Make?" (unpublished paper, Cape Town: arepp:Theatre for Life, 2006); Marian Nell & Janet Shapiro, "'Beyond Gut Feeling': Report on the arepp:Theatre for Life Evaluation Project 2002–2004" (unpublished evaluation; Cape Town: arepp: Theatre for Life, 2005).

[2] Lynn Dalrymple, "Has it made a difference? Understanding and measuring the impact of applied theatre with young people in the South African context," *Research in Drama Education* 11.2 (2006): 201–18; Bob Dick, *Qualitative action research: improving the rigour and economy* (1999), http://www.scu.edu.au/schools/gcm/ar/arp/rigour2.html (accessed 19 August 2008); Victoria J. Marsick, "Action Learning and Reflection in the Workplace," in *Fostering Critical Reflection in Adulthood: A Guide to Transformative and Emancipatory Learning*, ed. Jack Mezirow (San Francisco: Jossey–Bass, 1990): 23–46; Warren Parker, "The Development of Community-Based Media for AIDS Education and Prevention in South Africa: Towards an Action-based Participatory Research Model" (Masters thesis, University of Natal, Durban, 1994).

[3] Dalrymple, "Has it made a difference? Understanding and measuring the impact of applied theatre with young people in the South African context"; Dick, *Qualitative action research: improving the rigour and economy*; Marsick, "Action Learning and Reflection in the Workplace."

bringing about future change and, as such, is interventionist and particularly suited to development paradigms and discourses, particularly on health.[4]

Action research has roots in phenomenology and postmodernism, which validate experience as a valid way of knowing. Originating in Dewey's philosophical pragmatism, Lewin's social psychology, and Piaget's cognitive-developmental epistemology, and as initially popularized by Kolb,[5] the field of experiential learning examines how individuals and groups (primarily of adults) gain knowledge and make meaning from their direct, lived experience; positing that people learn from reflection, processing, challenging, and understanding what they personally do or experience.

> Learning may be defined as the process of making new or revised interpretation of the meaning of an experience, which guides subsequent understanding, appreciation, and action.[6]

Experiential learning's focus is on how the participant, either as an individual or as a collective, cognitively makes meaning from their experiences and how this produces knowledge – and what elements, determinants, and power relationships within the experience contribute to, influence, or impede that process.[7]

According to Jack Mezirow, learning from experience occurs in two forms: *instrumental learning*, in which people learn from engaging in task-orientated problem solving or learning from doing; and *communicative learning*, in which people learn from understanding the meanings of what others commu-

---

[4] *Qualitative action research: improving the rigour and economy*; B. Dick, *Action research: action and research* (2002), http://www.scu.edu.au/schools/gcm/ar/arp/aandr.html (accessed 19 August 2008).

[5] David A. Kolb, *Experiential Learning: Experience as the Source of Learning and Developmunt* (Englewood Cliffs NJ: Prentice–Hall, 1984), http://www.learningfromexperience.com/research-library/ (accessed 19 August 2008).

[6] Jack Mezirow, "How Critical Reflection Triggers Transformative Learning," in *Fostering Critical Reflection in Adulthood*, ed. Mezirow, 1.

[7] Tara Fenwick, "Expanding conceptions of experiential learning: a review of the five contemporary perspectives on cognition," *Adult Education Quarterly* 50.4 (2000): 243–72, and "Reclaiming and re-embodying experiential learning through complexity science," *Studies in the Education of Adults* 35.2 (2003): 123–41; Kolb, *Experiential Learning*; Mezirow, *Fostering Critical Reflection in Adulthood*; Elana Michelson, "Carnival, paranoia, and experiential learning," *Studies in the Education of Adults* 31.2 (1999): 140–54.

nicate "concerning values, ideals, feelings, moral decisions, and such concepts as freedom, justice, love, labour, autonomy, commitment and democracy"[8] or learning by interpreting. Understanding is achieved, then, by critically reflecting on the experience, either empirically or metaphorically. Kolb's experiential-learning theory proposes a cycle of learning which moves through four stages: the 'Concrete Experience', followed by 'Reflection' on that experience, which leads to theorizing on the experience ('Abstract Conceptualization') and, finally, to adaptation of the next experience ('Active Experimentation').[9] The processes of reflection, conceptualization, and adapted praxis can, however, be understood to be dynamically and fluidly linked and can occur simultaneously,[10] and the notion of cognitive reflection, analysis, and conceptualization can also be achieved through embodied, participatory, and contextual discourses with, and within, the experience.[11]

Experiential learning focuses on how people can best learn from their experiences. It is specifically participant-based, in the sense that it focuses on the people involved in the experience, either individually or collectively learning from that experience and putting that learning into practice. It is also both individual and social, in that the learning is considered in the social context of the experience and the other participants. As such, experiential learning is seen as occurring through discourse or in dialogue, as participants judge and validate meanings and assertions empirically.[12] Experiential learning is skills- and practice-based, as it focuses on enabling participants to process and learn from their experiences and to put that learning into practice. Experiential learning is thus, at its heart, transformative and emancipatory, making a

---

[8] Mezirow, "How Critical Reflection Triggers Transformative Learning," in *Fostering Critical Reflection in Adulthood*, ed. Mezirow, 8.

[9] J.S. Atherton, *Learning and Teaching: Experiential Learning* (2005), http://www.learningandteaching.info/learning/experience.htm (accessed 19 August 2008); Kolb, *Experiential Learning: Experience as the Source of Learning and Development* (Englewood Cliffs NJ: Prentice–Hall, 1984).

[10] Fenwick, "Reclaiming and re-embodying experiential learning through complexity science"; Mezirow, *Fostering Critical Reflection in Adulthood*; Michelson, Michelson, "Carnival, paranoia, and experiential learning."

[11] "Reclaiming and re-embodying experiential learning through complexity science"; "Carnival, paranoia, and experiential learning"; Gay Morris, "Practising role play: Learning through experience," *South African Theatre Journal* 19 (2005): 8–71.

[12] Mezirow, *Fostering Critical Reflection in Adulthood*; Michelson, "Carnival, paranoia, and experiential learning."

distinction between the performance of experience that is reinforcing, habitual and hegemonic, and critical reflection, reassessment, and learning followed by reflective, adapted, re-embodied action. Although the model as initially put forward by Kolb is highly cognitive and rational, current thought in experiential learning permits a variety of approaches and models; because experiential learning is practice-based and focused, it means that the practice or experience itself determines the best means of learning from it.[13]

Fenwick identifies five approaches to or perspectives on experiential learning, which she labels 'reflection', 'interference', 'participation', 'co-emergence', and 'resistance', each with a slightly different view of knowledge and learning, and each with a different perspective on the role and relationships between the participant, knowledge, and the context; however, all "share the assumption that certain experiences of cognition can be enhanced in ways that produce outcomes desired by the actors or learners involved."[14] In Fenwick's view, participants can learn from their experiences by coming to terms with and understanding the conflicts generated between the interference of their conscious thought by their unconscious desires; through the interaction between their participation and the context in which it occurs; through the emerging adaptation of themselves and the environment for their mutual coexistence; through determining the influences of the power hierarchies of race, gender, culture, ethnicity, ideology, and identity; and through the conscious and active review of, and reflection on, the experience.[15]

Fundamental to achieving experiential learning, however, is the fact that cognition occurs through some form of reflecting upon and engaging in discourse with the experience, its social context, and the other participants. 'Reflection' is used here not as Fenwick does to refer to a particular approach to cognition, but, rather, as an overarching term to define the act of cognitive engagement with the experience. Reflection is defined by Dewey as "assessing the grounds [justification] of one's beliefs"[16] and by David Boud as "a

[13] "Expanding conceptions of experiential learning: a review of the five contemporary perspectives on cognition"; "Reclaiming and re-embodying experiential learning through complexity science."

[14] "Expanding conceptions of experiential learning," 245.

[15] "Expanding conceptions of experiential learning"; "Reclaiming and re-embodying experiential learning through complexity science."

[16] Dewey, in Mezirow, "How Critical Reflection Triggers Transformative Learning," in *Fostering Critical Reflection in Adulthood*, ed. Mezirow, 5.

generic term for those intellectual and affective activities in which individuals engage to explore their experiences in order to lead to new understandings and appreciation."[17] The Oxford English Dictionary defines reflection as "the mode, operation, or faculty by which the mind has knowledge of itself and its operations, or by which it deals with the ideas received from sensation and perception."[18] Reflection should therefore not necessarily be seen as a separate cognitive and rational activity divorced from the experience, nor should meaning-making be separated from the process of experiencing or reflecting on the experience. As Fenwick states,

> reflection itself is experienced, and experience as event cannot be separated from our imaginative interpretation and re-interpretation of the event.[19]

Cognitive engagement with the experience is a fluid, generative, and continuous interaction in which the participant constantly moves between the frames of observer and participant seeking to understand the meaning of the experience. whether from a constructivist, a psychoanalytic, a situational, an enactivist, or a critical-cultural stance. Reflection should be seen as an act of self-reflexive engagement with an experience in order to learn from that experience; it is a mode of cognitive discourse with the experience that leads to transformation. Cognitive discourse determines the difference between simple repeated performance and adapted praxis. Reflection, whether connotative, analytical, participatory, or phenomenological, is the meaning-making activity whereby engaging with the experience becomes cognitive learning and forms the basic premise of the learning model of action research.

Action research encourages the use of any research methods, theories or approaches that can contribute to the understanding and improvement of the practice.[20] Based in the 'action-reflection' model of experiential learning, action research requires the involvement of the participants in the learning process, critically reflecting on their own practice in order to determine theory

---

[17] Boud, in Mezirow, "How Critical Reflection Triggers Transformative Learning," in *Fostering Critical Reflection in Adulthood*, ed. Mezirow, 5.

[18] *The Oxford English Dictionary*, Eleventh edition revised, ed. Catherine Soanes & Angus Stevenson (Oxford UP, 2006), *Oxford Reference Online*, http://www.oxfordreference.com (accessed 15 February 2008).

[19] "Reclaiming and re-embodying experiential learning through complexity science," 126.

[20] "Action Learning and Reflection in the Workplace."

and further develop praxis. Action research is thus firmly rooted in Freire's notion of critical pedagogy[21] and enabling people to reflect critically on their actions in order to change their circumstances and their praxis. Action learning

> is highly compatible with many of the premises on which adult education is built. It is driven by peers, focused on immediate problems, based on learner experience, and highly participatory.[22]

There are three key integrated components of the action-research process: action, reflection, and the development of theory.[23] These components are applied in an ongoing cyclical process, the rigour of which comes from the continuous testing and reviewing of practice. It is this cyclic, reflective, developmental approach that arepp:Theatre for Life has attempted to structure into a formal monitoring and evaluation system.

'After the Curtain' is the arepp:Theatre for Life procedure for assessing, monitoring, evaluating, and reporting on the productions and their impact – what the organization refers to as its "M&E system".[24] Through a continuous, ongoing process of testing, reflecting on, and adapting its practice, arepp: Theatre for Life has developed specific indicators for the presentations which attempt to capture the potential for the development of self-efficacy regarding the specific issues among audiences, and thus the impact of the projects. The design uses a grounded-theory type of approach to the data[25] and is similar to the methods expounded by Miles and Huberman for qualitative data collation, investigation, and analysis.

---

[21] Paulo Freire, *Pedagogy of the Oppressed*, tr. Myra Bergman Ramos (*Pedagogía del oprimido*, 1971; Harmondsworth: Penguin, 1972).

[22] "Action Learning and Reflection in the Workplace," 44.

[23] Dick, *Action research: action and research*; "Action Learning and Reflection in the Workplace,"

[24] arepp:TfL] arepp:Theatre for Life, "After the Curtain: Monitoring and Evaluation 2009," in *The Big Deal: arepp:Theatre for Life Performer's Training Manual* (unpublished document, Cape Town: arepp:Theatre for Life, 2008).

[25] Ian Dey, "Managing data," Creating categories," "Assigning categories," in Dey, *Qualitative Data Analysis: A User-Friendly Guide for Social Scientists* (London: Routledge, 1993): 77–86, 100–19, 120–36; Matthew B. Miles & A. Michael Huberman, "Early Steps in Analysis," in *Qualitative Data Analysis: An Expanded Handbook* (Thousand Oaks CA: Sage, 1994): 50–88.

The initial process of determining the impact indicators and the initial development of the system is detailed in "After the Curtain"[26] and was a continuous process of action and reflection on the meaning of impact in the arepp:Theatre for Life context and on finding ways to express that in a 'measurable' form. This process remains ongoing for the organization, and is reflected in annual adaptations and refinement of the system, as detailed in the 'Monitoring and Evaluation' section of the performance team's training manual.[27]

arepp:Theatre for Life defines its ethos or vision as

> a supportive society in which the individual members are active directors of their own lives, taking responsibility for making informed choices which lead to empowered decisions for their holistic growth. This, in turn, contributes to the constructive development of their society. The initiation and reinforcement of self-efficacy and resilience in individuals, groups and communities promotes a change in social attitudes, choices, behaviours and morés regarding sex, sexuality, relationships and gender, contributing to a reduction of the rates of HIV transmission, discrimination, human rights abuses, abuse, gender-based violence and rape, and thus the increased mental and physical health of society.[28]

In this context, arepp:Theatre for Life understands the impact of its applied-theatre presentations to be the following:

> the audiences will develop resilient self-efficacy and so be enabled with informed choice for sustainable decision-making with regard to sex, sexual and reproductive health, sexuality, and their relationship and life-style choices and behaviours in order to
> • make sound, informed lifestyle choices about what is best for them, and their community, in their particular contexts;
> • accept and take responsibility for those decisions;
> • and be flexible and robust in responding to the consequences, both foreseen and unforeseen.[29]

---

26 Bilbrough, "After the Curtain: Designing an Impact Monitoring and Evaluation System for an Edutainment Theatre Intervention."

27 "The Big Deal: arepp:Theatre for Life Performer's Training Manual" (unpublished document, Cape Town: arepp:Theatre for Life, 2008).

28 [arepp:TfL] arepp:Theatre for Life, "General Proposal 2009" (unpublished document, Cape Town: arepp:Theatre for Life, 2008): 5.

29 arepp:Theatre for Life, "General Proposal 2009," 5.

Self-efficacy is understood to be the perception, ability and competence of a person, group or community to understand, influence, change, and maintain their concept of themselves and their attitudes, beliefs, behaviours, values and life-style choices, and includes their capacity to be tolerant, flexible, and adaptable.

Resilience is the capacity of a person, group or community to respond to, transcend, withstand and recover from changes, setbacks or adversity.

The outcome that arepp:Theatre for Life therefore expects from each presentation is

> an increase in the perception, ability and competence of the audiences to understand, influence, change, adapt and maintain their concept of themselves and their own choices, attitudes, beliefs, behaviours, values and views with regard to their rights, HIV/AIDS, sexuality, gender equality and relationships, and in their acceptance and tolerance of the choices, attitudes, beliefs, behaviours, values and views of others.[30]

For a person to develop self-efficacy requires knowledge, awareness, and understanding of the self, the context, and the issues presented; and the skills, competency, belief, and problem-solving abilities to make and sustain decisions regarding them.[31]

The specific objectives of each arepp:Theatre for Life presentation are thus

> — To increase and develop the resilient self-efficacy of South African school-going youth in relation to sexuality and sexual and reproductive health issues through
> — the provision of relevant factual information,
> — increased knowledge of the self, the issues and the context,
> — the enforcement of a positive self-concept,
> — and the development of rights-based problem-solving and decision-making life-skills.[32]

Knowledge in this context is understood to be awareness and understanding of the information, attitudes, beliefs, behaviours, values and social norms pertaining to the issues presented.

---

[30] "General Proposal 2009," 5.

[31] Bilbrough, "Playing For Keeps: An examination of arepp:Theatre for Life's applied theatre pedagogy with regard to adolescent sexuality" (doctoral dissertation, University of Cape Town, 2009).

[32] "General Proposal 2009," 5.

Self-concept is understood to be the whole inner 'picture' that people have of themselves, including such traits as self-image, self-confidence, self-competence, self-value, and self-worth – how they think, believe, and feel about themselves.

Life-skills are understood to be the means whereby a person identifies, communicates, and solves problems, and makes and maintains decisions regarding their own attitudes, beliefs, modes of behaviour, values, and life-style choices.

The alignment of the presentations with the life-orientation curriculum ensures that each performance occurs within, and supports, each grade's syllabus work on these issues, providing educators with a resource and reference point for their annual life-orientation outcomes and assessment. In terms of the life-orientation curriculum, the impact of arepp:Theatre for Life is expressed in the following outcomes:

> CRITICAL OUTCOMES Learners are able to:
> CO 1: Identify and solve problems and make decisions using critical and creative thinking.
> CO 5: Communicate effectively.
> CO 6: Show responsibility towards the environment and the health of others.
> CO 7: Demonstrate an understanding of the world as a set of related systems by recognizing that problem solving contexts do not exist in isolation.
>
> SPECIFIC OUTCOMES Learners are able to:
> SO 1: Understand and accept themselves as unique and worthwhile human beings.
> SO 2: Use skills and display attitudes and values that improve relationships in family, peers and community.
> SO 3: Respect the right of people to hold personal beliefs and values.
> SO 4: Demonstrate value and respect for human rights.
> SO 5: Practice acquired life and decision-making skills.
> SO 7: Demonstrate the values and attitudes necessary for a healthy and balanced life-style.[33]

---

[33] Department of Education, *Curriculum 2005: Life Orientation Revised National Curriculum Statements Grades R to 12 (Schools) Policy* (Pretoria: Department of Education, 2003–2004).

The development of self-efficacy is not a single event but, rather, a process that occurs along a continuum. Impact is therefore also understood to occur at various places on this self-efficacy continuum to facilitate and support these outcomes – from a person's initial awareness, through facilitating the processes of choice and decision-making, to assisting in their maintenance – depending on where the person is in relation to the issue, their personal development, and their particular personal and life circumstances.

arepp:Theatre for Life has defined five *Self-Efficacy Indicators* to express this:

SPARKED AWARENESS: the stage at which a person becomes *aware*, where he or she was not hitherto, of possible choices regarding an attitude, a form of behaviour, a belief, a value.
REINFORCED UNDERSTANDING: the stage at which a person's *understanding* of the context, options, and consequences of an attitude, a form of behaviour, a belief, a value, is reinforced.
ENCOURAGED CHOICES: the stage at which a person *engages* with the possibilities and options of changing an attitude, a form of behaviour, a belief, a value for themselves.
SUPPORTED DECISIONS: the stage at which a person *changes* an attitude, a form of behaviour, a belief, a value.
VALIDATED LIFE-STYLES: the stage at which a person is supported in *living* and *maintaining* attitudes, forms of behaviour, beliefs, values.

arepp:Theatre for Life's applied-theatre pedagogy combines the concepts of observational learning through a theatre show with the processes of experiential learning through facilitated discussion, via the experience of a tailored theatrical 'event', to develop self-efficacy. The theatre experience stands in for and simultaneously transmogrifies into a life experience for the audience, which is then reflected upon, analysed, and theorized, and where skills are imparted to understand how to solve problems and make sense and meaning of experience.[34]

This development of self-efficacy is achieved through the engagement of the audience in the show and in the facilitated discussion afterwards. The better an arepp:Theatre for Life presentation succeeds in engaging with the

[34] Bilbrough, "Playing For Keeps."

audience, the greater the environment for, and likelihood of, an increase and development in that audience's self-efficacy.

The arepp:Theatre for Life method achieves this engagement via the processes of fostering identification, arresting empathy, and precipitating cognition so that the audience members experience 'themselves' reflected in and refracted through the prism of the event. The experience becomes a life experience for the audience, which, in turn, increases the reservoir of life experiences and competencies that the audience has to draw on when faced with and responding to real-life situations. The more of such opportunities or experiences that a person has in relation to the actions or forms of behaviour depicted, and the more skilled and able they are to analyse and interpret them, the more they will have to draw on to help them shape their actions and responses to actual life events, thus developing resilient self-efficacy.[35]

Accordingly, the level of an audience's engagement depends on the quality of the presentation, their personal identification and emotional involvement with the performance, their cognitive participation in the production and in the discussions and debate which follow, and the provision of relevant, rights-based information.

Identification is understood as a powerful feeling of affinity with the characters and their situations, and involves potentially regarding the characters as models that they may recognize, aspire to, or avoid; adopting, realizing or rejecting their attitudes, beliefs, forms of behaviour, life-styles, or values.

Cognition is the mental ability and process of acquiring knowledge regarding information, attitudes, beliefs, forms of behaviour, values, and social norms by the use of reasoning, intuition, or perception.

The monitoring and evaluation system has been designed to rigorously and systematically assess the engagement of the audience and record, by means of forms, the specific issues raised in order to determine the degree to which the presentations outcomes and their impact are likely to have been achieved.

Initially, during the selection and arrangement process with each school, the project staff collect a basic statistical profile of the school's learner complement in relation to size, gender, language, economic status, number of orphans and vulnerable children, National Senior Certificate pass-rates (secondary schools only), and reported incidents of sexual and physical abuse (including peer abuse/bullying), pregnancy, and suicide (including attempts).

[35] Bilbrough, "Playing For Keeps."

This provides a basic indication of the context in which the presentations will occur.

During the rehearsal process, each arepp:Theatre for Life performance team is trained to work with the various forms and assessment criteria that make up the system to assess critically and record the learners' reactions to and involvement in the performance, their participation in the facilitation sessions, the questions asked, and the discussions held, and then, in group discussion, to rate and report on their impressions of the audiences' engagement with the presentation, both quantitatively and qualitatively, to assist with later recall, discussion and reflection for reporting.

Once in performance, during the facilitation sessions the performance team records all the questions, and the substance of the subsequent discussion and debate, by gender and age-group focus on a 'Facilitation Discussion Record' form.

The team 'code' the questions in relation to the specific topics discussed from the spectrum of arepp:Theatre for Life content issues:

> Abuse, HIV/AIDS, Identity Issues, Rights & Responsibility, Relationships, Reproductive Health, Sex & Sexuality, Substance Use and Performing.

At the conclusion of each presentation, the arepp:Theatre for Life team assess the event using a 'Show Information & Assessment' form. The team describe their experience of the show and the audience, detailing anything unusual or particularly interesting. They then critically analyse and rate their impression of the audience's *engagement* with the presentation as a whole, using the following assessment criteria to inform their ratings

Assessment Criteria

The degree to which the audience

- responded and interacted appropriately during the performance;
- remembered and recounted the characters, situations and events of the play;
- related to the characters, situations and concerns;
- recognized and expressed problems they identified with or were grappling with themselves;
- discussed problem-solving techniques to find solutions;

recognized and discussed a range of options and their various consequences;
applied factual knowledge to problem-solving and decision-making processes;
discussed where to seek factual information and support;
displayed a willingness to accept responsibility for decisions and choices they discussed;
expressed ideas of where and how to exercise their rights in the context of the South African Constitution;
displayed a sense of worth, confidence, self-respect, and self-knowledge;
expressed tolerance of alternate choices, beliefs, modes of behaviour, life-styles, and views.

Engagement Indicators

Response: the audience responded appropriately;
Information: the audience were (re)informed with relevant factual information;
Identification: the audience personally identified with the characters and situations;
Involvement: the audience were emotionally involved with the production;
Cognition: the audience cognitively participated in discussion and debate about the issues.

Each of the engagement indicators is rated on a four-point scale with the options 'not at all', 'partially', 'well', and 'exceptionally well'; where 'not at all' has a value of 1 and 'exceptionally well' a value of 4. The team supports their ratings with a narrative paragraph that summarizes their impressions of the audience and explains their choices using examples from the show and the discussion. Based on this, the team also suggests possible areas for further follow-up and support.

The life-orientation educators and two learners, one of each gender, also assess and evaluate each presentation, by means of assessment questionnaires, for comparison and analysis.

The life-orientation educators are asked to rate the audience's *engagement*, using almost the same engagement indicators, and in the same way on the 'Educator's Evaluation' form, which they are given before the show begins. For the educators, however, the 'response' indicator is replaced with the following 'information' indicator, as the educators would not know what an appropriate response might be but are able to assess the relevance of the information provided. For the educators, the word 'learners' also replaces 'audience'.

Information: The learners were (re-)informed with relevant factual information.

In addition, the educators rate the quality of the show and the facilitation session, and the degree of relevance of the presentation to the life-orientation curriculum. The educators then evaluate the demonstrated and expected increase in the life-skills of the audience based on their training, experience, and knowledge of their learners, and their observations during the presentation, using the *Life-Skills Indicators*, which are drawn from the life-orientation curriculum outcomes.

Life-Skills Curriculum Indicators

Communication: increase in the learners' ability to communicate effectively;

Problem-solving: increase in the learners' ability to identify and solve problems and make decisions;

Skills: Increase in the learners' use of skills and display of attitudes and values for improving themselves and their relationships with family, peers, and community;

Choices: support of the learners' values and attitudes for healthy and balanced life-style choices and modes of behaviour;

Rights: increase in the learners' demonstrated respect for the right of people to hold personal beliefs and values and their rights;

Responsibility: increase in the learners' demonstrated responsibility towards themselves, their peers, their community, and their society.

Each of the life-skills indicators is rated on the same four-point scale with the options 'not at all', 'partially', 'well', and 'exceptionally well'; where 'not at all' has a value of 1 and 'exceptionally well' a value of 4. As with the team, the educators then support their quantitative ratings with a qualitative comment on their impressions of the effect on the audience, and share their views on the possible long-term impact of the presentations. A team member ensures that the evaluation is completed immediately after the presentation so that it can be collected and to answer and record any questions the educator may have.

Immediately after the presentation, the team select two learners, one from each gender and from the same grade, to complete the relevant 'Learner's Evaluation' form (with the foundation-phase learners, the performers ask the questions and record their answers). The choice of learners is as random as possible, and throughout the process of the tour the team attempt to provide a balance between the ages, grades, and perceived degree of involvement of the members chosen to represent the full spectrum of the audiences. For ethical reasons and to satisfy full disclosure, the team member explains that the evaluation form is used to assist arepp:Theatre for Life in monitoring, assessing, and improving the shows, that it is anonymous, and that it may be used in arepp:Theatre for Life's reports.

The learners rate their engagement by rating their feelings on the following *Experience Indicator Statements* using a four-point scale with the options 'not at all', 'a little', 'yes', and 'a lot'; where 'not at all' has a value of 1 and 'a lot' a value of 4. These are used to rate the learners' *engagement* with the experience. Like the educators, they also rate the quality of the show and the discussion, and are asked to share their feelings or thoughts qualitatively about the show and the discussion afterwards and what it meant to them.

Learners' Experience Indicator Statements

The statements in italics are not given to the intermediate-phase learners (grade 4 to 7).

- *The play felt like real life to me.*
- The play held my interest.
- *Things like this happen in my school.*
- I responded to the characters and their stories.
- My feelings were touched by the play.
- I felt comfortable with the discussion.
- *I trusted the facilitators of the discussion.*
- I felt free to ask my questions in the discussion.
- I learnt something from the presentation.
- The presentation relates to what I've been learning in Life Orientation.
- *I trusted the information presented.*

- I understood the information presented.
- I know where to find more information if I want to.

The learners also rate their perception of their self-efficacy after the production on the self-efficacy continuum by indicating whether they 'agree', 'disagree', or are 'not sure' which of the *Self-Efficacy Indicator Statements* apply to their experience of the presentation.

Self-Efficacy Indicators

Sparked Awareness: I learnt about and saw some things in a new way;
Reinforced Understanding: it reminded me of what I already knew, felt and understood about some things;
Encouraged Choices: I feel like making some changes to the way I do some things or how I think about them;
Supported Decisions: I believe I can change the way I think, feel and behave about these things if I want or need to;
Validated Life-Styles: I am happy, comfortable with and feel supported in the choices I have already made about these things.

The self-efficacy statements indicate the audiences' perception of their feelings of competence, agency, and self-worth in relation to the issues after the presentations – their perceived self-efficacy.

A team member remains with the learner(s) completing the evaluation so that it can be collected and to answer and record any questions the learners may have.

The *Foundation phase* learners (grade 1 to 3) are asked the following questions:

- How did you feel about the play, was it (tick) Bad/OK/Good/Excellent & Why?
- What did you like most about the play? Why?
- What didn't you like about the play? Why?
- What did you learn?
- Is there anything else you would like to tell us?

At the end of each day, the team goes through all the forms for each show as a group to confirm and enhance their general impression of the day. They ensure that all the details are correct, and they enter the data in the Microsoft Excel 'Tour File' spreadsheet provided for that purpose.

The intention is to capture the experience of each presentation with each individual audience. In this way arepp:Theatre for Life attempts to determine where in relation to the development of self-efficacy each audience appears to be sited with regard to the main issues that were relevant to them from each presentation, and what potential areas may need additional concentration, follow-up or support.

At the end of each tour, arepp:Theatre for Life then compiles and captures each individual presentations' assessments into the aforementioned 'Tour Report', which reflects an analysis of the level and nature of the engagement and the interaction of the audiences with the production, in order to gain an impression of the potential impact on the audience's self-efficacy. The performance team remind themselves and reflect on the tour by taking the completed 'Show Information and Facilitation Discussion Record' forms and highlighting examples that represent the overall quantitative ratings calculated in the Excel 'Tour File', are a good reflection of the average/general/common responses, comments, and questions, as well as all negative comments, suggestions or problems, using the following coding:

RED – NEGATIVE/PROBLEMS
GREEN – POSITIVE/IMPACT
BLUE – SUGGESTIONS/REQUESTS

Simultaneously, the project staff do the same with the 'Educators' and Learners' Evaluations'.

Once all the shows have been assessed a meeting is held with all relevant staff to reflect on the tour, after which the 'Tour Report' is written following an established format, reporting on all key indicators.

'Formal Narrative Reports' regarding the status of the project, the various shows, and the tours are then produced quarterly, detailing these assessments, with an 'Annual Narrative Report' to summarize on a yearly basis. All these reports attempt to summarize, inform about, and track changes in attitudes, trends, and perceived self-efficacy.

In this way, arepp:Theatre for Life records, monitors, and assesses the presentations and their audiences. The assessments are tracked and compared with the situations, environments, and profiles gathered from other presentations and other schools. This enables arepp:Theatre for Life, over time, to demonstrate changes in the knowledge, attitudes, belief, skills, and values of the audiences regarding the issues, and the development of their self-efficacy, and thus the impact of the project.

For example, the graph below reflects an increase in those learners who completed evaluations perception of their feelings of competence, agency, and control over the issues invoked for them by the presentations, clearly indicating a shift 'down' the self-efficacy continuum towards making choices, and taking control and responsibility over decisions, over the three years 2006 to 2008. arepp:Theatre for Life considers this to be a clear indication of an increase in the self-efficacy of the learners over the period, especially when understood on the basis of the fact that 50% of the schools engaged with an arepp:Theatre for Life presentation repeatedly – that is, once each year for the three years – during the period.

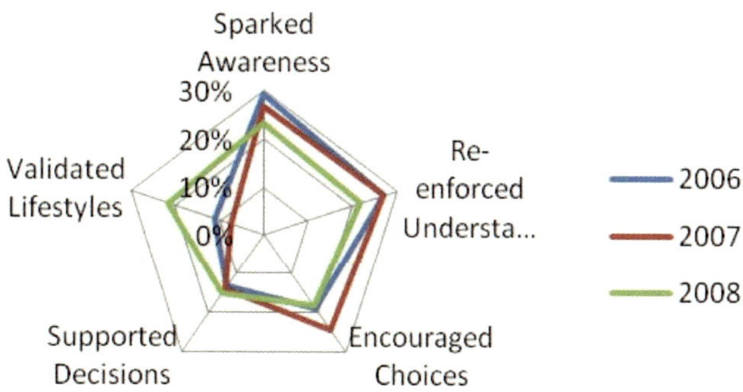

Figure 1: Learning increase, 2006–2008[36]

In the arepp:Theatre for Life context, this cyclical, reflective, developmental approach has had a profound effect on the development of the organization and its methodology, leading to an increased depth and understanding of how the applied-theatre presentations work, the impact that they have, and how to monitor, assess, and evaluate that impact. Thus it is that the organization has made certain fundamental changes to methodology, content and approach over the years, moving from 'Puppets Against AIDS' and adult HIV/AIDS education to Theatre for Life and the development of decision-making and problem-solving life-skills and self-efficacy among learners in schools. In the

[36] arepp:Theatre for Life, "1st Quarter 2009 Narrative Report" (unpublished document, Cape Town: arepp:Theatre for Life, 2009): 10.

context of HIV and AIDS, where the impact of applied-theatre interventions is often difficult to demonstrate, this has proven to be invaluable.

The Forms

The forms which 'operationalize' this system and capture the data are as follows:

The 'Show Information & Assessment Form'
The 'Facilitation Discussion Record'
The 'Educator's Evaluation'
The 'Learner's Evaluation' (per age-group focus: foundation, intermediate, senior)
The Microsoft Excel 'Tour Files' spreadsheet.

Works Cited

[arepp:TfL] arepp:Theatre for Life. "After the Curtain: Monitoring and Evaluation 2009," in "The Big Deal: arepp:Theatre for Life Performer's Training Manual" (unpublished document, Cape Town: arepp:Theatre for Life, 2008).

[arepp:TfL] arepp:Theatre for Life. "General Proposal 2009" (unpublished document, Cape Town: arepp:Theatre for Life, 2008).

[arepp:TfL] arepp:Theatre for Life. "The Big Deal: arepp:Theatre for Life Performer's Training Manual" (unpublished document, Cape Town: arepp:Theatre for Life, 2008).

[arepp:TfL] arepp:Theatre for Life. "1st Quarter 2009 Narrative Report" (unpublished document, Cape Town: arepp:Theatre for Life, 2009).

Atherton, James S. *Learning and Teaching: Experiential Learning* (2005), http://www .learningandteaching.info/learning/experience.htm (accessed 19 August 2008).

Bilbrough, Gordon. "After the Curtain: Designing an Impact Monitoring and Evaluation System for an Edutainment Theatre Intervention" (unpublished report, arepp: Theatre for Life: Cape Town, 2004).

——. "Playing For Keeps: An examination of arepp:Theatre for Life's applied theatre pedagogy with regard to adolescent sexuality" (doctoral dissertation, University of Cape Town, 2009).

——. "What Difference Does It Make?" (unpublished paper, Cape Town: arepp: Theatre for Life, 2006).

——, & Brigid Schutz. "From Puppets Against AIDS to Theatre for Life" (unpublished paper, Cape Town: arepp:Theatre for Life, 2006).

Dalrymple, Lynn. "Has it made a difference? Understanding and measuring the impact of applied theatre with young people in the South African context," *Research in Drama Education* 11.2 (2006): 201–18.

Department of Education. *Curriculum 2005: Life Orientation Revised National Curriculum Statements Grades R to 12 (Schools) Policy* (Pretoria: Department of Education, 2003–2004).

Dey, Ian. "Managing data," Creating categories," "Assigning categories," in Dey, *Qualitative Data Analysis: A User-Friendly Guide for Social Scientists* (London: Routledge, 1993): 77–86, 100–19, 120–36.

Dick, Bob. *Action Research: Action and Research* (2002), http://www.scu.edu.au/schools/gcm/ar/arp/aandr.html (accessed 19 August 2008).

——. *Qualitative action research: improving the rigour and economy* (1999), http://www.scu.edu.au/schools/gcm/ar/arp/rigour2.html (accessed 19 August 2008).

Fenwick, Tara. "Expanding conceptions of experiential learning: a review of the five contemporary perspectives on cognition," *Adult Education Quarterly* 50.4 (2000): 243–72.

——. "Reclaiming and re-embodying experiential learning through complexity science," *Studies in the Education of Adults* 35.2 (2003): 123–41.

Freire, Paulo. *Pedagogy of the Oppressed*, tr. Myra Bergman Ramos (*Pedagogía del oprimido*, 1971; Harmondsworth: Penguin, 1972).

Glaser, Barney G. *Basics of Grounded Theory Analysis* (Mill Valley CA: Sociology Press, 1992).

Kolb, David A. *Experiential Learning: Experience as the Source of Learning and Development* (Englewood Cliffs NJ: Prentice–Hall, 1984), http://www.learningfromexperience.com/research-library/ (accessed 19 August 2008).

Marsick, Victoria J. "Action Learning and Reflection in the Workplace," in *Fostering Critical Reflection in Adulthood: A Guide to Transformative and Emancipatory Learning*, ed. Jack Mezirow (San Francisco: Jossey–Bass, 1990): 23–46.

Mezirow, Jack. "How Critical Reflection Triggers Transformative Learning," in *Fostering Critical Reflection in Adulthood: A Guide to Transformative and Emancipatory LearningFostering Critical Reflection in Adulthood: A Guide to Transformative and Emancipatory Learning*, ed. Mezirow (San Francisco: Jossey–Bass, 1990): 1–20.

——. *Fostering Critical Reflection in Adulthood: A Guide to Transformative and Emancipatory LearningFostering Critical Reflection in Adulthood: A Guide to Transformative and Emancipatory Learning* (San Francisco: Jossey–Bass, 1990).

Michelson, Elana. "Carnival, paranoia, and experiential learning," *Studies in the Education of Adults* 31.2 (1999): 140–54.

Miles, Matthew B., & A. Michael Huberman. "Early Steps in Analysis," in *Qualitative Data Analysis: An Expanded Handbook* (Thousand Oaks CA: Sage, 1994): 50–88.

Morris, Gay. "Practising role play: Learning through experience," *South African Theatre Journal* 19 (2005): 8–71.

Nell, Marian, & Janet Shapiro. *"Beyond Gut Feeling": Report on the arepp:Theatre for Life Evaluation Project 2002–2004* (unpublished evaluation; Cape Town: arepp: Theatre for Life, 2005).

The Oxford English Dictionary, ed. Catherine Soanes & Angus Stevenson (Oxford UP, 11th rev. ed. 2006). *Oxford Reference Online* (Oxford University Press, University of Cape Town), http://www.oxfordreference.com (accessed 15 February 2008).

Parker, Warren. "The Development of Community-Based Media for AIDS Education and Prevention in South Africa: Towards an Action-Based Participatory Research Model" (Master's thesis, University of Natal, Durban, 1994).

⌘

REBECCA ANN RUGG

Collaboration as Research

Yale University, Siwela Sonke Dance Theatre, Clowns Without Borders South Africa, and People's Educational Theatre Swaziland

THIS ESSAY DESCRIBES AN EVOLVING MODEL for artistic and pedagogical collaboration through interdisciplinary, multi-institutional, intercultural practice. Through it, I hope to offer one approach to a research paradigm appropriate for applied drama and theatre. The answer proposed here is that artistic collaboration itself is a research paradigm, and the ways in which we structure collaboration are a methodology, a grammar of research. In proposing this, I am in good scholarly and artistic company – practitioners know well that the ways we make art are a means to understanding the world – including questions of who leads and who follows, how we share leadership in the rehearsal room and onstage. From Richard Schechner to Patrice Pavis,[1] significant thinking has been done on the subject; particularly excellent is recent work of the theorists Jacqueline Lo and Helen Gilbert, who analyse multiple methodologies of international collaboration, finding in

---

[1] Richard Schechner, *The End of Humanism: Writings on Performance* (New York: Performing Arts Journal, 1982), and "Interculturalism and the Culture of Choice: Richard Schechner Interviewed by Patrice Pavis," in *The Intercultural Performance Reader*, ed. Patrice Pavis (London: Routledge. 1996): 41–50; Patrice Pavis, *Theatre at the Crossroads of Culture* (London: Routledge, 1992), and "Introduction: Towards a Theory of Interculturalism and Theatre," in *The Intercultural Performance Reader*, ed. Patrice Pavis (London: Routledge, 1996): 1–19.

some examples the means to denaturalize the "universalist vision of the more egregious kinds of interculturalism."[2] Lo and Gilbert seek collaborative methods that provide "pathways into intercultural projects that resist an unproblematized transfer of culture";[3] this, too, is an ambition of the project I'll describe here. In attempting to create an intercultural collaboration mindful to multidirectional cultural flows and a keen awareness of power relations, it was thus both an artistic and research project.

In using collaboration itself as a research paradigm, I also draw heavily on the work of Paolo Freire, whose brilliant reconception of teaching as learning has offered a powerful example of re-orientation. As we are familiar, in Freire's pedagogy, teaching is a transitive process, a dialogue, where it is only possible to teach someone who teaches in return. Augusto Boal says of his mentor:

> With Paulo Freire, we learned to learn. In his method [...] one learns to know and to respect otherness and the other, difference and the different. My fellow creature resembles me, but he is not me; he is similar to me, I resemble him. By engaging in dialogue we learn, the two of us gain, teacher and pupil, since we are all pupils, and all teachers. I exist because they exist.[4]

As in teaching, where the outcome of a class may ultimately be the students' possession of new knowledge but the process of getting there may be the most important and illuminating aspect of the experience, the process of artistic collaboration may end most obviously in performance, but along the way often offers other kinds of challenges and exchanges that may productively be understood as research results.

Importantly, this focus on the structures of collaborative process re-orients what Osita Okagbu has called "the existential imperative of Theatre for Development which is, exist to transform the audience into makers and owners of the theatre event and experience."[5] In the project I'll describe here, the

---

[2] Jaqueline Lo & Helen Gilbert, "Toward a Topography of Cross-Cultural Theatre Praxis," *Drama Review* 46.3 (Fall 2002): 31–53.

[3] Lo & Gilbert, "Toward a Topography of Cross-Cultural Theatre Praxis," 20.

[4] Augusto Boal, "Paulo Freire, my last father," in Boal, *Legislative Theatre: Using Performance to Make Theatre*, tr. Adrian Jackson (*Teatro legislativo*; London & New York: Routledge, 1998): 129.

[5] Osita Okagbu, "Product or Process: Theatre for Development in Africa," in *African Theatre for Development*, ed. Kamal Salhi (Exeter: Intellect, 1998): 24.

primary focus was on the methods of collaborating to create applied theatre across cultures, which meant that the subjects of the event were the artists themselves and not their prospective audiences; put another way, the artists were their own community and audience, and the project provided time for self-reflection and attempting new methods. While not responsive to the important practical goals of theatre for development or applied theatre, this focus may in turn offer a new perspective on the process of collaboration with audiences as makers of the theatre experience.

It is through the framework of these ideas that I'll now describe an evolving collaboration that took place in Swaziland and South Africa from 2007 to 2009. In June 2007, I inaugurated an interdisciplinary course whose most explicit goal was to introduce undergraduates from Yale, the university where I teach in the USA, to major issues of the HIV/AIDS pandemic in southern Africa through the dual perspectives of public health and applied theatrical practice. In each of three years, the course design built on the outcomes of the previous year's collaboration. In 2009, the course involved a project with Durban's acclaimed Siwela Sonke dance theatre, and in Swaziland, a joint collaboration with Clowns Without Borders South Africa and People's Educational Theatre. The essay will describe some of the outcomes and challenges for the various stakeholders across the three years of the project – local artists, public-health and theatre faculty, students. It will also consider central questions of developing an intercultural model of collaboration and pedagogy.

This has been a project undertaken from the USA, where my primary work is as a theatre producer, dramaturg, and educator; because many US practitioners are underexposed to international practice, sometimes at home describing the challenges and successes of this project has been difficult. Navigating the different vocabularies of US community-based theatre practice, academic discussion of intercultural work, and the history of political understandings of theatre for development and applied theatre in the global South is often quite difficult. To some degree, the varied vocabulary in the field reflects a healthy interdisciplinarity of the work being undertaken. Amidst this healthy variety, I aim to be clear in my own descriptive vocabulary, but am also aware that nomenclature often carries historical weight that may perhaps be invisible to me as an outsider.

I Impulse and Inspiration

My own inspiration for undertaking this course derives from coming of age during the early days of the AIDS crisis in the USA, and my peripheral but personally significant exposure to the direct action group ACTUP New York, the AIDS Coalition to Unleash Power, which was how I discovered theatre, and where I first understood the powerful potential of the theatrical gesture in civil society. As I've become a theatre professional and scholar, I have heard repeatedly from US artists that they have a desire to be doing more influential work than creating art. My early exposure to direct-action politics has convinced me that the struggle to assert the social impact of art is not merely an expression of insecurity on the part of individual artists but, rather, part of a systemic problem. Of course, it is not unique to the USA that the arts are undervalued, and that artists have trouble maintaining their belief in the social importance of their work – the anti-theatrical prejudice is alive and well in many corners of the globe. But it is also true in the USA that aspiring artists have access to multiple opportunities for education and training – really, an over-abundance of training programmes – and yet are often deeply uncertain of their social relevance and impact in culture.

An opportunity to attend the World Social Forum in Nairobi in 2007 expanded my thinking on these ideas. As part of an international artist delegation, I had the opportunity to hear from African artists at the convention about a desire for training, and a widespread frustration with commissions from non-governmental organizations or other socially invested groups driving the content of their work. However, even amidst this frustration, the artists we encountered seemed to be in touch with the deep purpose and meaning of making art. Within this personal history and context, I became motivated to ask how it might be possible to offer an experience of obviously influential artistic practice to US culture workers. Together with this, how would it be possible to offer resources of training and new techniques to artists abroad, particularly in the Global South, while learning techniques and ideas about social uses from them in a sound and mutually beneficial model? These new questions added to ongoing lifelong questions: How can we use art to stop AIDS? How can art be used for healing?

II Moving Forward/2007

I teach at Yale School of Drama, an elite graduate theatre training conservatory in the US. Yale has vast resources, and is a seat of cultural privilege and power. For me, the politics of working in a place like this demand active advocacy to direct resources to artists and to projects that wouldn't otherwise have them. In working to create space for intercultural collaboration in this context, with this funding arrangement, I understand that whatever is ultimately created will necessarily be mediated through US economics, driven by a Western vision of exchange in ways that may only become visible to me over time. I discussed my idea for intercultural artistic collaboration funded by the University with two colleagues who share similar passions, Ntare Mwine and Gamal Palmer, both artists trained as actors, working in multiple media. After we put together a proposal, I sought a home for it in a variety of different areas of the University, including the graduate school in which I'm primarily appointed. While the University at large avows its commitment to 'globalizing' education, and the individuals whom I approached were enthusiastic about the project, all were uncertain as to where resources might be found. After significant institutional legwork, I found one haven, inside the office of the Yale Summer Session, a fairly autonomous department with progressive, forward-thinking administrators. Under these auspices, we were able to move quickly forward with a version of the project that was implemented as a course for undergraduates during Yale's 2007 June Summer Session.

In the first year of the course, I led a faculty team composed of Professor Kaveh Khoshnood, from Yale's School of Public Health, the US/Ugandan artist Ntare Mwine as Master Artist, Gamal Palmer as graduate teaching assistant, and Meredith Coleman–Tobias, a graduate student from Yale's Divinity School accompanying as a researcher. Over the course of a month's residency with twenty Yale undergraduates in Swaziland, we did short multi-day workshops with six different theatre companies. We experienced the work of each of these companies in performance, and then discussed and heard about their histories and missions; after that, Mwine led workshops on a variety of theatrical techniques for the artists and students together. We also met with various non-theatre groups, including a support group for people living with HIV/AIDS, an underground progressive political party, and a collective of grandmothers running a neighbourhood care point. In this first year, we elected to organize the schedule so as to give as broad a view as possible of Swazi theatre and culture to students, and to expose them to as many different companies of artists as possible – for the US faculty, this also provided an overview and an opportunity to meet and find like-minded collaborators for future years, since there had not been much time on the ground in Swaziland to organize the course initially.

Over the course of a month's work with this variety of groups, Professor Khoshnood gave lectures to joint groups of Yale students and Swazi artists about what epidemiologists call the 'natural history' of HIV, by which is meant the progress of the disease within the body, and on other scientific topics relevant to the epidemic. This proved to be useful, and in some cases new information for artists who were working to convey vital information about the disease to audiences. In discussions I led, I counteracted the notion of the 'natural history' of HIV, which I thought made the epidemic sound inevitable, by offering a cultural and performative history of the epidemic, particularly of the gross political neglect that occurred during the early days in the USA. As a discipline, public health follows what Freire called a banking model of education, and aspires to a kind of neutrality in its reliance on statistics – whereas, in my teaching, I am used to showing my cards politically. I teach a history in which I was involved, and about which I have passionate views. In this disciplinary gap between the theatre historian and the epidemiologist, Mwine conducted several workshops for groups of artists and students – for instance, on mask-making out of locally found materials. In this work, Professor Khoshnood was very much open to participating in several theatre exercises, which created strong channels of communication between him and the Swazi artists.

From several different theatre companies, we learned of the heavy international aid presence in Swaziland, and noticed a kind of fatigue among artists at being called upon to make socially engaged work. In fact, there was a kind of culture-wide AIDS fatigue. Or, even more than fatigue, it began to seem that many people we met were in a state resembling shock. We had originally planned to work in Swaziland because it is the country with the highest incidence rate of HIV/AIDS in the world, which seemed a good reason to put resources there, and to contribute to what positive work was being done there to stop the epidemic. These reasons did not sit well with the Swazi artists we encountered that summer. As a whole, they disliked the attention devoted to Swaziland for the reasons of the epidemic – while, at the same time, displaying an ironic awareness of the ways in which international aid provides some economic opportunity for certain Swazis. Despite – or perhaps because of – this astute political analysis, and its accompanying gallows humour, the Swazi artists we met would rather people come to Swaziland because it is beautiful and because of their wonderful culture, of which they are very proud.

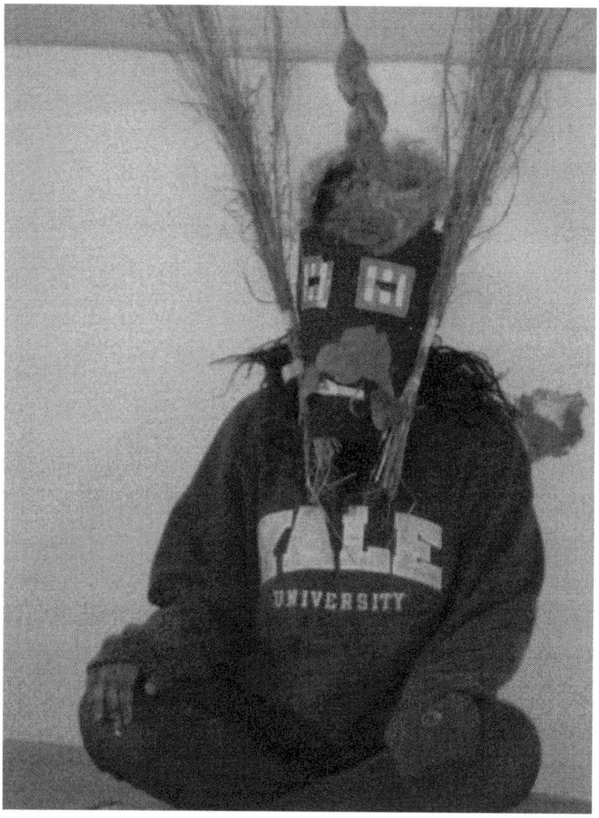

Figure 1: Student with project mask

In assessing the first year of the project, which in some ways was very successful, it was clear that several things had been missing, and many questions had not been asked. Assessment in this first year took the form of my documenting the activities we had undertaken, and then soliciting evaluations in conversation with each of the faculty individually. There was a shared sense that we had not created a depth of connection between Swazi artists and Yale students, partly because we worked with several different groups of artists over the course of our time in the country, and also because the Swazi artists had not been in leadership roles.

Other issues in the assessment included language and venue. In setting up the course, I hadn't understood (and still do not fully) how English functions relative to SiSwati in common speech among regular people in Swaziland; and how linguistic power dynamics function in communication with speakers of US English. As Lo and Gilbert observe,

> An elementary but immensely important question is the matter of whose language is used for everyday communication during the devising and rehearsing of specific productions. The fact that English has become the lingua franca in an increasingly globalized arts community gives its native speakers considerable power to substantiate their views and/or secure their particular agendas. [...] To ask whose values are heard and whose are silenced by the use of specific languages therefore seems essential to a more politicized form of interculturalism.[6]

An entire, extremely productive inquiry could focus on this particular aspect of intercultural collaboration; our realization after one month's residency was that the widespread assurance we had received that Swazi people spoke English with total fluency was itself a political statement, reflecting the desire for this to be true and erasing the complex regional, economic, and cultural reasons why it was not always the case. In terms of space, we had similar questions after the initial year of the project. Reflecting upon the multiple venues in which our work had taken place, clearly the choice of meeting places had inflected the work created, but in exactly what ways remained opaque; consequently, so did how best to move forward.

Some goals came clearly into focus after just a month of intensive time with artists and undergraduates in Swaziland. For the students, the experience, if constructed correctly, had the power to encourage them to question and encounter openly; to learn experientially; to have a deep commitment to people unlike themselves; and to think very carefully about the dynamics at work in their relationships with people across difference. However, the model we had employed in this initial year, of bringing a master-artist with the Yale team and placing him in a position of leadership over the Yale students and Swazi artists alike, had not been conducive to this kind of open encounter, since the workshops were overly constrained by time, and thus fairly regimented. I had questions about what kinds of leadership might better serve the collaboration, and also about what might be the benefits for the local artists. Out of exploratory conversations with Swazi artists, the first year's experiences yielded a set

---

[6] Lo & Gilbert, "Toward a Topography of Cross-Cultural Theatre Praxis," 46.

of broad questions: How might it be possible to set up an annual, short-term programme that would benefit local artists and their local communities? Or, at the very least, would do no harm, and not function to drain existing resources? How would it be possible to bring resources that could support local artists and organizations to do more of what they're already doing, rather than enforcing an external agenda? Or, conversely, how could the resources of this course give artists the chance to do something that they otherwise might not have the resources to do?

III Re-Orienting/2008

In our first year, we had worked with People's Educational Theatre for several days, and had felt a strong sense of connection to these artists. In part, this was because their work was spectacular and varied – we saw them perform a kind of Forum Theatre piece on spousal abuse in a rural community centre, part of a programme of Swaziland Action Group Against Abuse (SWAGAA), and also a high-paced traditional dance show at a dinner celebration. I was interested to learn more about how they understood their work in various vocabularies of theatre, ranging from applied to entertainment-driven. Several outspoken individuals among the group had also been quite impressive in their willingness, during group discussions, to question our motives at being in their country, and, further, to probe what we intended to do with what we learned when we returned home. These were good conversations, prompting questions, and we were glad to have found a group of people who were ready to speak their mind and state contrary opinions. I recognize that these aspects of our communication may have appealed to my own culturally American orientation towards informality and candour; this sensibility was a primary force in moving towards further collaboration with this group.

Therefore, in the second year of the course, we undertook a longer collaboration with PET while in Swaziland, aiming to achieve a greater depth of connection. We also planned this year to split our time between Swaziland and Cape Town, in order to collaborate with the South African Tuberculosis Vaccine Initiative, learning about this project, and providing theatre workshops for the public-health workers. This was an effort to provide a more in-depth experience of public-health work for the students, within one of the most forward-thinking and ethically sound vaccine trials in the world. Because of this in-depth public-health project, the faculty team was reconfigured so that we were without a US public-health scholar, but instead there were two theatre professionals, and a graduate teaching assistant from Yale's Divinity School, Meredith Coleman–Tobias, who had accompanied the project the year before in an informal capacity, pursuing her own research on the connections between spirituality and theatrical practice in the region. Based on her work in the previous year, it was clear that she would be an invaluable resource to the faculty team, particularly in helping the students navigate some of the more emotionally and spiritually challenging aspects of being in a country in the midst of a public-health crisis.

In planning, primarily via email, for the section of the course to take place in Swaziland, I suggested a model where one lead artist from PET, Nicholas Mamba, would work jointly with my co-teacher, Gamal Palmer, to produce a performance in which Yale students and Swazi artists acted together. In retrospect, it is clear that the suggestion of shared leadership was not explored fully enough prior to our arrival – and that, despite the quality of candour of the Swazi artists, they might not have felt they could suggest alternatives once I had brought up this model of collaboration. I had a lot to learn (and surely still do) about the kinds of power that were at work in our conversations, but that were invisible to me.

Another alteration to the course in its second year, this one more successful, was that it began for the Yale students with a week in New Haven, rather than the Yale group's travelling to meet for the first time in Swaziland. In this way, the students were able to begin with classroom learning about topics in public health, and move into more experiential learning once abroad. During this week, one main goal was to re-orient students to understand that they were going to Southern Africa to learn rather than to 'help'. Their impulse tended to be precisely the opposite, for several understandable reasons, including a desire to take responsibility for the economic benefits many of them possess, and their inculcation in an educational system that prizes leadership above all. Convincing these students to allow themselves to learn and not spring prematurely into action is quite difficult.

One activity that was very successful in this re-orientation was an evening of 'culture-sharing', in which each member of the class – including faculty – shares a cultural practice based on familial, ethnic, racial, regional or some other affiliation entirely. Often the 'culture' students choose to share is located in bodily practices – that year, two students from Pakistan and India taught us Bangra dance, and two others from Detroit taught us the Ballroom Hustle. Lo and Gilbert describe intercultural exchange as being on a continuum, one end of which they characterize as "imperialistic," which "is often driven by a sense of Western culture as bankrupt and in need of invigoration from the non-West."[7] The evening of culture-sharing with the class was an attempt to get us away from this side of the continuum; in learning from each other, it became clear that the vector was not about travelling to experience 'authentic culture' elsewhere, in a kind of tourist orientation, but carrying cultural knowledge and diversity within the group which we could share with fellow artists. When the Swazi artists met the group on their arrival in Swaziland, then, and shared song and dance with them in a circle, the students were prepared, and had some moves of their own to contribute.

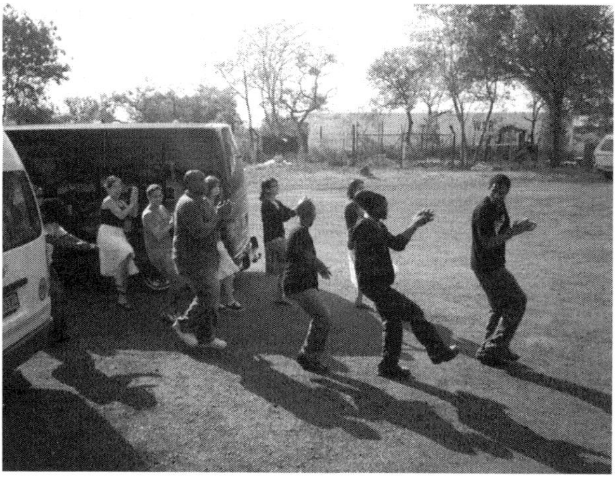

Figure 2: First-encounter dance

Some of the challenges in this second year included the US faculty team's discovering that an aspiration for shared leadership – which may have been one-sided to begin with – revolves around an understanding of devised work which is common in the USA but not in Swaziland. It is obvious, but worth stating, that leadership in different cultures is performed differently. One common model for shared leadership in theatrical collaboration in the USA is to alternate exercises or parts of rehearsal, with different people leading. We were struck by how different this is from always trying to forge joint decisions, which is what we observed the Swazi artists doing in the circle. That summer, the Yale group came to appreciate, though probably not fully understand, the radical equality of the circle, with its rotating leadership, at times

[7] Lo & Gilbert, "Toward a Topography of Cross-Cultural Theatre Praxis," 39.

planned and, at others, based on the impulse of the moment. This is crucially different from a pre-planned model of back-and-forth shared leadership. A longer, very productive study could be made of the different kinds of artistic process and results that each model achieves.

This year, as with the first year, much of our rehearsal happened at the Mbabane Theatre Club, which we rented. This building is the only purpose-built theatre in Swaziland, and is a leftover from the days of the British protectorate, when it housed locally produced versions of canonical Western plays, and also touring shows. It is now fairly run-down, and also houses a small restaurant and daycare operation on its grounds, ways by which the ownership attempts to find income, since the theatre is not often used for performances. Rehearsal in this building often sprawled onto the lawn outside or into the lobby, which transformed the theatre temporarily into an informal space – however, there was a certain built-in formality to the architecture that may have inhibited fully free exploration. Certainly, when exercises happened outside, movement was more expansive, choices bigger, and laughter louder. Lo and Gilbert suggest one very good question to ask with regard to the spatial aspect of intercultural collaboration: "Whose ground are we on?"[8] Noticing the differences in the work made inside and outside of the Theatre Club, I was aware of how its architecture and its concomitant history were constituting our collaborations in space – this space didn't belong to any of us who were in it, and in fact had been designed precisely to alienate certain constituencies.

The show created by PET artists and the Yale students began with the circular warm-up they had all been practising together – this was an effort to help the Yale students, many of whom were new performers, with anxiety, and also out of a shared desire to begin inside the shape we had discussed so much. The play was a journey story around discovery of a treatment for HIV, with the protagonist role shared between a Yale student, Brandon Wheatley, and the PET member Stanley Mabuza (Figure 3), and a guiding storyteller figure as well, played by the PET member Musawenkosi Zikalala (Figure 4). It was performed only twice – at a high school and in the nKwalini neighbourhood where Zikalala lived. At the school, it seemed to be a source of confusion and subsequent interest that there were black members of the Yale contingent, including Wheatley, who shared the protagonist role with Mabuza.

[8] Lo & Gilbert, "Toward a Topography of Cross-Cultural Theatre Praxis," 47.

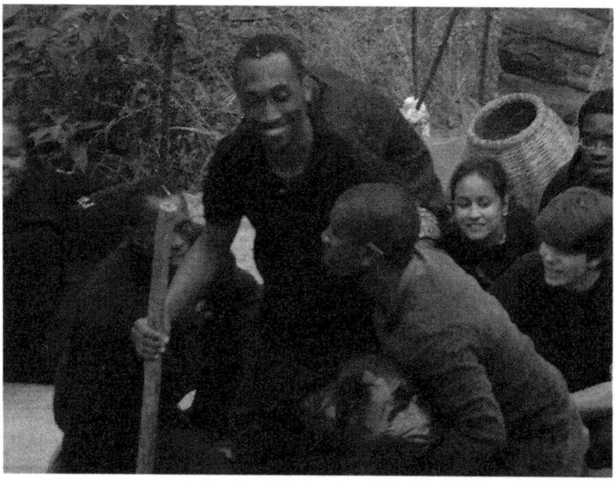

Figure 3: Brandon Wheatley and Stanley Mabuza

The show's performance in nKwalini, a community just outside of downtown Mbabane, was prompted by an extraordinary undertaking on the part of Musa Zikalala. The year before, Gamal Palmer had frequently visited the Zikalala family homestead in nKwalini, and had returned full of stories about this family, and about the theatre which Zikalala had begun to create on their hill-side. When we decided to work with PET again the next year, one of our hopes was to be able to support Zikalala's completion of this theatre. The very existence of this theatre is fascinating, given the restriction on civil assembly in Swaziland, which has been in effect since 1973, prohibiting all forms of public discourse not expressly sanctioned by the King. Theatre, in this environment, is effectively illegal, though clearly there is much theatre activity taking place. However, it places artists in a precarious position, watchful over the content of their words and actions onstage. In this context, Zikalala's desire to build a theatre in his neighbourhood, as a gathering-place for local youth to learn Swazi traditions and to have something to do, was a radical act – not to mention the fact that creating a theatre singlehandedly in any context is a fairly radical proposition. Particularly impressive is the theatre project's arising out of Zikalala's own artistic impulses – in addition to dancing, acting, and drumming, he creates clothing, furniture, and paintings, and is an all-round talent, not observing any limitations of specialty. Here was a project that had nothing to do with what NGOs were telling Swazis to do to save themselves; but had everything to do with a lived-in understanding of the challenges facing people – the need for a place to gather to have fun, and to learn about their culture intergenerationally.

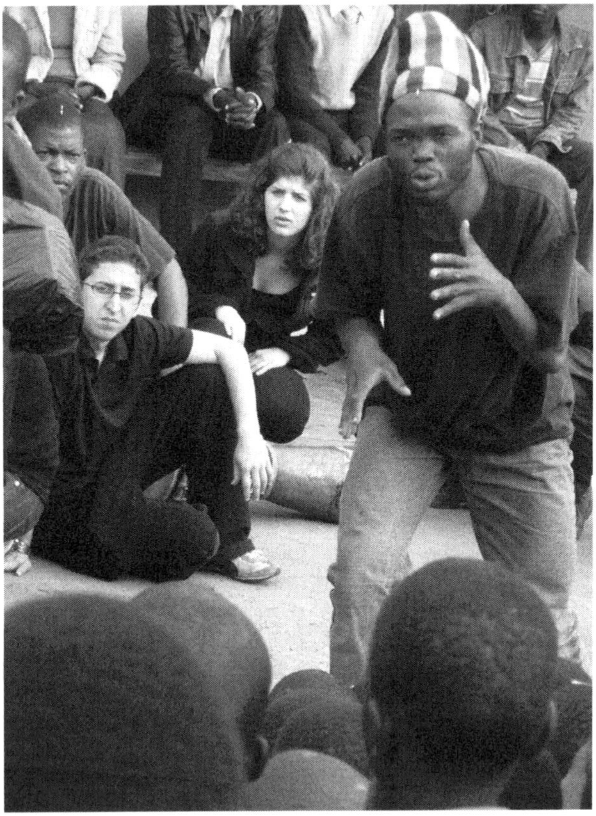

Figure 4: Storyteller figure played by Musawenkosi Zikalala

Zikalala did finish his theatre that summer, after months of digging out what basically amounted to the side of a small mountain. He created there what can rightly be claimed to be one of the most beautiful theatres in the world (Figure 5). On the day of the performance, Zikalala's mother and the women in his family prepared a feast from a cow slaughtered for the occasion of inaugurating the new space. Yale resources went to support the feast and also the theatre's completion, which ultimately was a funding rather than artistically collaborative contribution. And yet, because our group worked together and was involved artistically, the ways in which Yale funding supported the whole collaboration – with salary and travel money for the artists, for instance – wasn't benefactorial in a removed or impersonal way. Certainly it was not funding in service of an outside agenda – at least, not beyond the agenda of our working together – since here the funds supported a building project that a Swazi artist had begun on his own, and a feast that was also the idea and request of the artists. While the theatre company and students rehearsed on the hillside, the community gathered over the course of the day, and saw that the Yale group and PET were making something together.

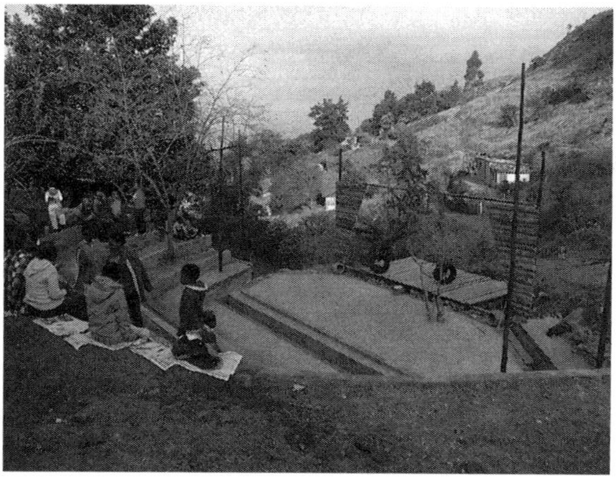

Figure 5: Musa Zikalala's theatre at nKwalini

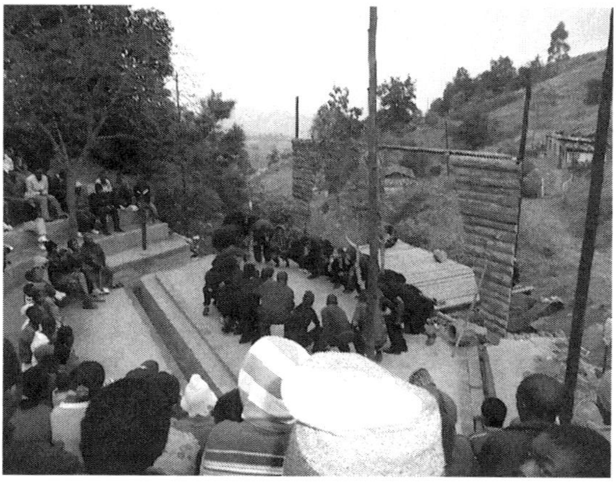

Figure 6: Rehearsal at nKwalini's hillside theatre

Eventually, the theatre was packed with men, women, and children, and the show and following feast were received with all the fervour of a major stadium concert, followed by torch-lit Swazi dancing and drumming. For me as a theatre professional, it was one of the most invigorating evenings I have ever spent in the presence of an audience. As a teacher, I saw and later heard directly how the Yale students felt themselves transformed by this embodied experience of community. What might come of this for each of them is open to time, something I'll look forward to finding out in the coming years. Personally, I was overcome with a feeling of gratitude to be invited into a community not my own, having as high an artistic experience as anyone could ever hope to have. Here, we had a new answer to the question 'whose ground are we on?' I want to be clear that I'm not making grand claims for the show we collaborated on, which was somewhat uneven in terms of quality – although that evening's performance showed the piece at its very best. Rather, I attribute the evening's success to the new theatre and the local community gathering. The venue offers PET the possibility to bring together all their skills as practitioners, from dancing to more character-driven theatre. This combination will forge a connection between elements of ritual and narrative to create or perhaps mend what Zodwa Motsa has called the "missing link"[9] in siSwati modern drama. That night, as theatre gave way to dancing, it was clear that this place could become a truly national and yet also importantly local home for contemporary Swazi theatre.

Assessment of the programme following this second year again yielded new questions and opportunities to alter and attempt to improve the shape of the collaboration. The assessment activities this year were somewhat more formal than in the previous year: each faculty member individually provided to me written documentation of the course's work, and then we met as a group two months after the course to discuss these documents in person; I conducted email discussion with members of PET, which was unfortunately quite spotty, and finally I synthesized these findings into one document for the University administration. In my own report following the programme in 2008, the evening I've just described didn't sit well with my received ideas about the responsibility of applied theatre to make lasting change, and I questioned whether the resources put towards one night's feast were well used. Importantly, this question did not seem to trouble our local collaborators at all, who had requested the feast and slaughter of the cow as a part of Swazi

---

[9] Zodwa Motsa, "The Missing Link in siSwati Modern Drama," in *Pre-Colonial and Post-Colonial Drama and Theatre in Africa*, ed. Lokangaka Losambe & Devi Sarinjeive (Cape Town: New Africa, 2001): 32–47.

tradition in honouring their ancestors in inaugurating a new community space. Perhaps in helping to provide this gift to the community, we had simply observed good manners as guests; in this, we would have been following in a centuries-long custom of what my mentor Joseph Roach calls "sacrificial expenditure," the often culturally complex performance of violence (hopefully, in this case, only to the slaughtered cow) for an audience in service of establishing culture and sustaining community.[10] After much pondering of how this event could be described as data, it was clear that while it would be difficult to articulate to a more regular foundation or NGO funding source how one meal for 500 people and one very enjoyable evening might make lasting change, what was liberating about doing this programme with undergraduates was that it was very easy to make the argument to the educational institution in favour of supporting a culminating artistic and cultural experience as being crucial to their learning.

In this second year of the course, we made huge improvements in the educational experience for the Yale students. We successfully created a schedule where they had adequate time to discuss and reflect upon the experiences they were having in and out of rehearsal, so that they were able to articulate their experience as learning, whereas, in the previous year, there had not been enough time for reflection. Much of the discussion had to do with questions of how to connect with others – their fellow students and African artists – across cultural, racial, and other lines of difference. We had set up enough of a trusting group dynamic in our first week in New Haven that these discussions were very open and deep, which was very encouraging. The programme in 2008 also answered some of the questions about what the benefits might be for local artists. In particular, the completion and inauguration of the nKwalini theatre promised to have lasting benefits both for the artists and the local community, and this had happened without the Yale group's enforcing an external agenda.

However, we had not productively answered the question of how to work collaboratively. The process of making the piece together had been frustrating and fraught with miscommunication about leadership, in particular. On several days, when the Yale faculty group had thought that the Swazi artists would be leading the work, they arrived unprepared and very late, and, on their side, the process of devising a piece out of small-group exercises was

[10] Joseph Roach, *Cities of* the *Dead: Circum-Atlantic Performance* (New York: Columbia UP, 1996): 41.

unfamiliar and not one that they were comfortable leading. We had not found a common language in this regard. If the length of collaboration each year were to remain a mere two or three weeks, I feared that it would be impossible to build a shared artistic vocabulary. While our ultimate showing of the piece had provided a positive experience of performance, the process had not been such a success. In this context, I returned to initial questions driving the project: how could the resources of this course give artists the chance to do something that they otherwise might not have the wherewithal to carry out? How might it be possible to leave these artists with new tools, or new relationships? How it might be possible for them to leverage the connection with Yale to their benefit in their own country?

IV Refining/2009

In planning for the third year of the course, I was interested in attempting a different model for the students' direct engagement with issues of public health. While the theatre-based work tended to prompt wide-ranging discussions about the nature of health and exposed the students to the lived perspectives of artists working on the ground floor of the pandemic, the students were eager for more exposure to traditional data and epidemiology. Over two years of the course, it had attracted a significant percentage of students whose professional goals lay in medicine, and, to my thinking, it was crucial to expose them to an analysis of health-care from the progressive point of view of community-based practice. To this end, I engaged as a faculty member Elizabeth Magenheimer, a nurse practitioner, to lead students on an investigation of a variety of clinical settings in our various travels, beginning with her own workplace, Fair Haven Community Health Clinic. Beginning there was strategic; it had become increasingly important to me that the students understand that there was extreme poverty and inequity in Yale's backyard; to understand that one important reason for the travel offered in this class was to begin to understand home differently.

Through a connection forged by the course faculty member Gamal Palmer, we had the opportunity in 2009 to work in Durban with the choreographer Jay Pather's world-class dance company Siwela Sonke. The company's mission is to use intercultural performance to break down historical barriers, and to tell the stories of people whose stories have not been told; our hope was that exploring a cross-cultural collaboration with this company would challenge students to understand health as it relates to a broad cultural fabric and history. After some frustrations in previous years around language, translation, and interpretation, the prospect of working with dancers in a physically based vocabulary was particularly interesting; and, indeed, the residency in Durban began with movement exercises, which brought the mixed company into communication without spoken language.

After two weeks of ensemble-building and dance classes, the group moved in two days to a quick process of creating short dance pieces, based on interviews conducted by pairs of Yale students and dancers. On the streets in downtown Durban, the pairs interviewed passers-by about the topic of "secrets." We had arrived at this topic out of conversations about how important the things are that people don't say or admit: this is true in thinking about public health and the HIV/AIDS pandemic, but also more broadly. The students and dancers made these interviews into poetry – took lines from the interviews and literally made poetry out of them, by abstracting and repeating phrases; then made poetry into dance – very abstract, beautiful shapes; and, finally, took these dances into public space, performing in downtown Durban (Figures 7 and 8). It was a tutorial in choreography with an aesthetic of fracture and rhythm, rather than message. This collaborative process showed the students and our faculty group how dance as a discipline is open to uncertainty in meaning, and how it has resisted the managerial language of 'outcomes', 'transparency', and 'messaging' that has become prevalent in theatre, particularly applied theatre. The Siwela dancers freely and appropriately claimed semiotic territory for art without explicit messages to be understood as topical material about HIV/AIDS, and about public health.

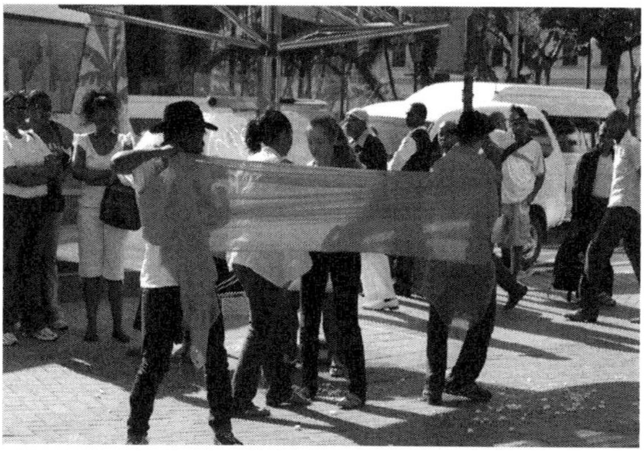

Figure 7: Street theatre, Durban

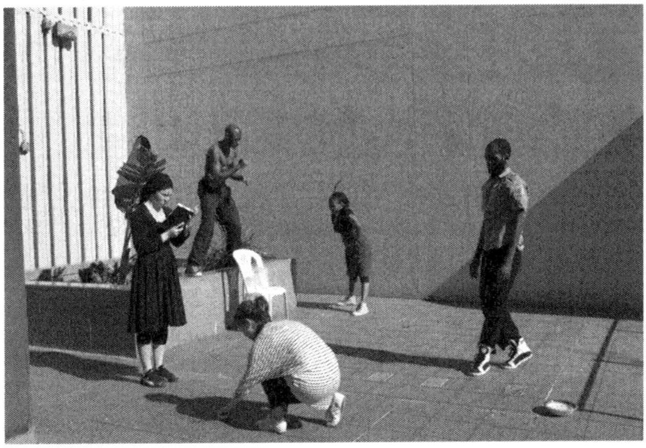

Figure 8: Street theatre, Durban

Questions driving this new collaboration with Siwela Sonke, from a faculty perspective, included: how to bring these world-class dancers into collaboration with world-class undergraduate students who are not (for the most part) trained in movement? What were the potential benefits for both parties? Clearly, the students weren't going to become dancers in two weeks, and the dancers weren't going to participate in all the reading and discussion outside of rehearsal that the students were doing. One answer to these questions was found in the pieces that were created, which were ephemeral, urban performances, jointly performed by small mixed groups of dancers and students. The dancers reported that they re-experienced their own city anew through the interviews and performances, especially through hearing and experiencing the students' questions; the students' reported that they had a completely different experience of Durban because of their connections to local people, rather than feeling only that they saw through foreign eyes. In this aspect, our work began to approach an intercultural experience that could be described as having a two-way flow, with all participants acting as cultural sources, rather than one group acting as sources of expertise.

Additionally, Siwela organized the rehearsals so that all dancers participating had opportunities to teach, something not normally the case, which provided them with experience leading the room. And the dancers did become students in the traditional classroom sense during several guest lectures, including one I gave on the history of AIDS and AIDS activism in the USA; they responded with surprise to find that this history in the USA was different from, and preceded, the pandemic in their country. When the Yale group went to visit McCord Clinic – a private hospital in Durban, with a significant apartheid-era history of treating Zulu patients – our visit there initiated a conversation among the members of the the joint company about access to health-care in the KwaZulu–Natal region, and in South Africa generally – something that probably would not have come up without the clinic visit, and provided perspectives on the politics of health-care that the students would not have gained without the process of artistic collaboration with Siwela. For the mixed company, complex ideas about health began to arise as a result of dancing and talking about the issue of "secrets."

After two weeks in Durban, the Yale group travelled to Swaziland. The pevious year, we had been fortunate to see a culminating performance of a project by Clowns Without Borders South Africa, a Durban-based group that often works in Swaziland, and had found both the performance and the articulated goals of the company to be compelling. Their work in using the body as a tool to provide laughter and healing was an exception in an environment where most applied theatre was for the purpose conveying information or promoting behavioural change. In this context, the work of Clowns Without Borders is refreshing, and provided a new avenue of performance research. CWBSA performs clown shows at schools, with their tagline 'no child without a smile' as one articulated goal, but also, together with community partners, the company undertakes longer-term healing initiatives with children and their guardians. These take the form of after-school workshops for playing theatre games – building resilience through drama, play, storytelling, creative movement, circus arts, and mindfulness-based stress relief. In conversation with CWBSA about a collaboration in 2009, it became clear that the company was eager to connect with Swazi artists, and also that Yale funds and participation could help support a follow-up residency for a programme the company had begun the year before.

Upon arriving in Swaziland, Yale students, together with our ongoing partners in PET, undertook one intensive week of clown training with the CWBSA master clowns in Swaziland's capital city, followed by another week of the follow-up residency, which involved performing clown shows and providing after-school workshops in Swaziland's rural south. My aim with this triangulated partnership was to connect the two groups – CWBSA and PET – through their participation in the course, in the hope of seeding a more long-term collaboration between them. CWBSA is well-connected within Swaziland to funding sources and local community partners, which could be shared productively with PET. Additionally, the collaboration promised to expose the artists of PET to a new, potentially profitable, and also eminently adaptable set of skills – physical theatre, which they could use or not, however they wished, in their future work. The idea for this collaboration returned to one of my root impulses for the course, which was to provide access to training to artists in resource-poor situations.

In the planning phase, I parted ways with a faculty member who objected to the plan for this three-way collaboration, Meredith Coleman–Tobias, who argued that trying to connect the PET artists with Clowns Without Borders was implicitly corrective and devalued the work of PET. Clowning, this line of thinking argues, is a Western form whose use in this context represented an act of cultural imperialism. She argued that we should return to do another piece with PET on the model of the previous year, and continue to explore the difficult territory of shared leadership, collaborative language, and the particular spiritual meanings of Swazi theatre. This perspective was strongly compelling, and troubling; however, it is crucial in the process of politicizing collaboration not to become paralyzed by ideas that suggest no kind of exchange can be ethical.[11] It was difficult to turn away from the initial exploration and potential discoveries of shared leadership in creating devised work with PET. However, my experience with collaborative matchmaking in professional theatre led me to believe that pursuing further the model we had used the year before had little hope of success, mainly because of the course's time constraints. Were we to have a year's, or even several month's, residency in Swaziland to collaborate with PET, it seemed to me that we might have a chance of success in creating an ethical, intercultural collaboration towards devising work; but, as it was, I chose what appeared to me to be the solution with the best chance of success, which offered many potential benefits to the Swazi artists, and in which they themselves expressed interest.

Students who took the course in 2009 experienced an embodied comparison between the physical work of clowning and contemporary dance. The connections they made with the Siwela dancers were friendly and warm; in Swaziland, however, since the two groups of African artists – PET and CWBSA – connected quite strongly, the students were to some extent excluded. Still, the sometimes terrifying experience of performing before hundreds of grade-school children was bonding for all the performers, Swazi, Zulu, and Yale students alike.

[11] Lo & Gilbert, "Toward a Topography of Cross-Cultural Theatre Praxis," 41.

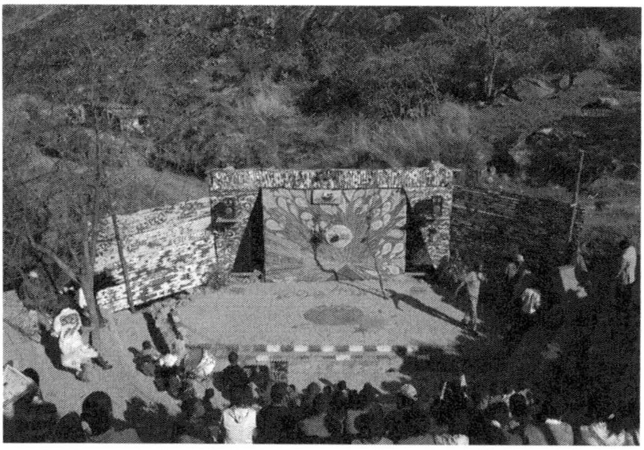

Figure 9: Musa Zikalala's theatre at nKwalini

This year, the resources of Yale benefitted the performers, but also the schools for which we performed, and children and guardians with whom we did workshops. Additionally, we performed the clown show at Zikalala's theatre in nKwalini on the night before we left, which had been further decorated and finished, and in just one year had become a vibrant centre for youth in the neighbourhood (Figure 9). As in the previous year, the performance was accompanied by a meal, and provided an enjoyable evening and experience of extraordinary community for the Yale students (Figures 10 and 11).

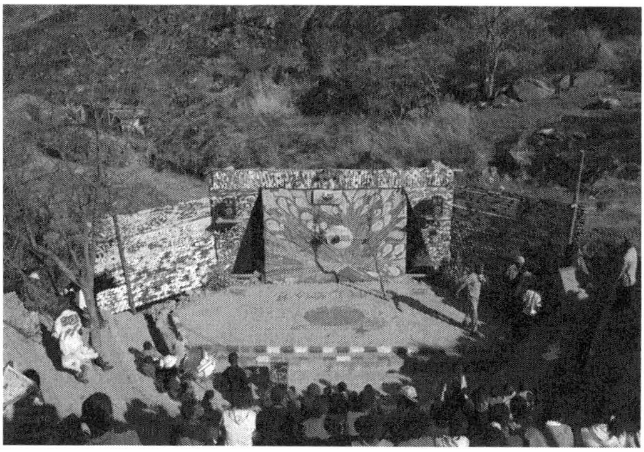

Figure 10: Performance at nKwalini theatre

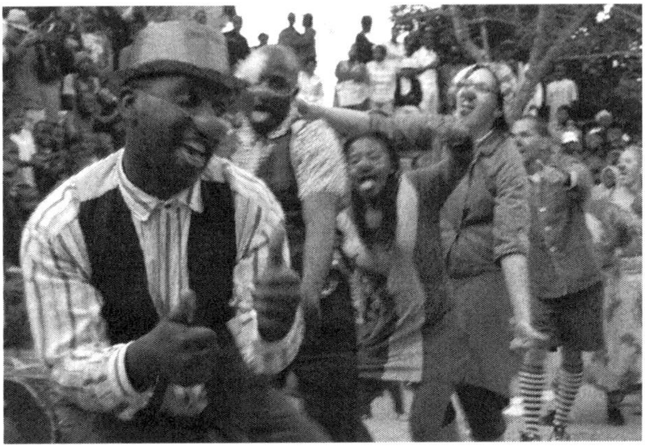

Figure 11: Clowning at nKwalini theatre

Since the programme, the PET artists have received opportunities to do what is perhaps the most difficult performing of all: clinic clowning, for children and sick people, in several hospitals in Swaziland; they have collaborated again with CWBSA, and, organizationally, CWBSA is training PET in grant-writing and involving the Swazi artists in a large scale UNICEF-funded roll-out of their intervention and residency programme in Swaziland. PET's artistic director had a fantastic residency at Yale, where he lectured and led seminars, his trip sponsored by the Divinity School and arranged by Meredith Coleman–Tobias. These practical outcomes allow me to believe that the programme over the years may have created an "intentional hybridity," something Lo and Gilbert locate at the opposite end of the spectrum of intercultural collaboration from imperialism;[12] which in this case enabled the navigation of multiple points of view, and the serving of multiple different needs on the part of very different participants.

V Closing

When this project found its home initially in the offices of the Yale Summer Session, I was glad to move forward but also somewhat ambivalent, since it meant that the work would take place with highly privileged nineteen- and twenty-year-olds, in collaboration with professional artists in Southern Africa,

[12] "Toward a Topography of Cross-Cultural Theatre Praxis," 45.

rather than with professional artists from the USA and their counterparts abroad, as had been my initial inspiration. The first year of the course was a kind of test model, upon which I embarked to see if it might evolve into what I originally intended. In other words, I thought at first that the class was the mechanism for something else.

After three years, the model has revealed itself to be deeply interesting in its own right. On one level, the project is an interdisciplinary study-abroad course in theatre and public health for undergraduates studying at Yale University. As I've described, challenges at this level include re-orienting a student mind-set which seeks to 'help' others toward a willingness to learn; organizing a faculty team from disparate disciplines – public health, dramaturgy, and acting – and gaining understanding of the complex issues involved in applied-theatre practice, which seeks to transform a culture of HIV/AIDS stigma into one of health and tolerance. At another level, the project seeks to bring the resources of this US educational institution to Southern African artists involved in socially engaged theatre and dance. The questions and challenges at this level are also vast: What kinds of leadership structures work best to facilitate interdisciplinary-intercultural collaboration? How should the duration of exchange and partnership affect the model of collaboration? In what ways may this collaboration be useful to local artists and the constituencies they serve? It has been the most challenging pedagogical journey I have undertaken as a teacher, attempting to lead a faculty team across disciplinary lines, handle group logistical matters in foreign countries, manage collaborative relationships with artists across lines of culture, race, and hemisphere, and at the same time to teach the undergraduate students, and analyse the experiences as research.

The challenges and questions above have served as gateways for research inquiries into pedagogy, theatre production, aesthetic practice, and interdisciplinarity. In this regard, the course and the encounters it provides serve both as practice and as research, and I report the initial steps towards founding the programme, the ongoing changes to the collaborative model, and my growing sense of the project's value as research outcomes. Each year, we begin the course by writing questions that will frame the coming experience; and, at the end of the course, create new framing questions based on what we have learned, and what we need to remember and consider upon returning home. This pedagogical practice reflects the idea that collaboration as research leads us not toward answers, but to better and better questions; it is my hope that, in reporting the refinement of my own questions about this project over time, they might be of use to others considering similar work.

WORKS CITED

Boal, Augusto. "Paulo Freire, my last father," in Boal, *Legislative Theatre: Using Performance to Make Theatre*, tr. Adrian Jackson (*Teatro legislativo*; London & New York: Routledge, 1998): 126–29.

Lo, Jacqueline, & Helen Gilbert. "Toward a Topography of Cross-Cultural Theatre Praxis," *Drama Review* 46.3 (Fall 2002): 31–53.

Motsa, Zodwa. "The Missing Link in siSwati Modern Drama," in *Pre-Colonial and Post-Colonial Drama and Theatre in Africa*, ed. Lokangaka Losambe & Devi Sarinjeive (Cape Town: New Africa, 2001): 32–47.

Okagbu, Osita. "Product or Process: Theatre for Development in Africa," in *African Theatre for Development*, ed. Kamal Salhi (Exeter: Intellect, 1998): 23–41.

Pavis, Patrice. "Introduction: Towards a Theory of Interculturalism and Theatre," in *The Intercultural Performance Reader*, ed. Patrice Pavis (London: Routledge, 1996): 1–19.

——. *Theatre at the Crossroads of Culture* (London: Routledge, 1992).

Roach, Joseph. *Cities of* the *Dead: Circum-Atlantic Performance* (New York: Columbia UP, 1996).

Schechner, Richard. *The End of Humanism: Writings on Performance* (New York: Performing Arts Journal, 1982).

——. "Interculturalism and the Culture of Choice: Richard Schechner Interviewed by Patrice Pavis," in *The Intercultural Performance Reader*, ed. Patrice Pavis (London: Routledge. 1996): 41–50.

⌘

NEHEMIAH CHIVANDIKWA

Participatory Theatre for Development as Action Research

Methodological, Theoretical and Ethical Challenges, Tensions and Possibilities with Specific Reference to an HIV/AIDS and Disability Project (2007–2010)

Introduction and Background

THIS ESSAY IS BASED ON A LARGER PROJECT on 'Disability and Empowerment in Participatory Theatre for Development'.[1] The present article focuses on HIV/AIDS and sexuality, which is one of the aspects covered. The essay discusses challenges and possibilities of interdisciplinary approaches in HIV/AIDS communication in the context of people living with physical impairments. Methodologically, the exploration is grounded in action research, whose practical processes are comparable and in most cases similar to participatory theatre-for-development processes. In fact, one of the key observations to be made in this study is that it is very curious and surprising that in Zimbabwe there has not been an attempt to relate research processes in theatre for development to key methodological and theoretical considerations in action research. I will submit that it will be beneficial if theatre-for-development practitioners appropriate key techniques from action research, particularly in addressing sensitive and emotive issues such as HIV/AIDS and sexuality among people with physical impairments. Closely

[1] The project is being carried out at the University of Zimbabwe under the broad theme: A Chosen Generation.

linked to the need to apply action research techniques in TfD practices is the desire to explore interdisciplinary approaches in the analytical frameworks of the exploration of HIV/AIDS themes in the context of people living with physical impairments.

The project under study began in 2007, involving myself and undergraduate applied-theatre students as animators. We discussed with officials and students from the University Disability Resource Centre (DRC) some of the challenges people with physical impairments face at the institution. However, it was later decided that the project should not just focus on local problems such as access to teaching facilities, recreational opportunities, and other academic and social discriminatory practices facing university students with physical disabilities. As a result, the project focuses broadly on social, political, and cultural barriers that deny physically challenged students access to resources, opportunities, and fundamental human rights in general. In order to emphasize the importance of inclusivity and active participation of affected groups, the project has embraced the popular motto 'Nothing About Us Without Us'. Each year, since 2007, a performance focuses on a specific major theme. At the time of writing, the major area of concern was HIV/AIDS and sexuality.

An artistic and participatory workshop held in August 2007 to create storylines became the basis on which participants interwove their personal experiences and observations with fictional narratives to collectively craft scenarios that challenge taboos and myths surrounding HIV/AIDS and sexuality as they related to people with physical impairments (see Appendix 1). Three such myths are worth mentioning here. The first myth is that people with physical impairments are asexual. This myth is dangerous, as it can complicate the spread of HIV/AIDS in addition to denying people with disabilities their full humanity. Second, the scenarios created confront the myth that visually-impaired women are 'competent' and extremely 'exciting' in bed or in love-making. The third is perhaps the most perverse, as it suggests that one can be 'cured' of HIV/AIDS through having sexual relations with people living with physical impairments. Generally, all the myths are based on discrimination, oppression, and superstition. These myths, once chosen, were then embellished and expressed through performance elements such as dramatic conflict, movement, sound, gesture, and voice to create fictionalized accounts of everyday realities facing people with physical disabilities.

Methodological Considerations

As already mentioned, the methodology adopted in this project is action research. This is a participatory approach to data collection, which is an essential component of in-depth emancipatory research. It is a process of dialogue, action, analysis, and change.[2] Action research is liberatory and transformative.[3] Knowledge in this methodological paradigm involves both the pedagogy of the oppressed and the pedagogy of the oppressor.[4] In this regard, self-learning is also crucial to researchers and practitioners. As a result, both myself and the students are using action-research techniques as a "common sense approach to personal and professional development that enables practitioners to investigate and evaluate their work and to create their own theories of practices."[5] In short, one deploys action research to improve practice and to generate new "theories," since action research is partly practical theorizing, with theory and practice transforming continuously into each other in a seamless flow.[6]

There are two major groups involved in this project. On the one hand, we have myself and applied-theatre students as animators of the project, officials who are mostly social scientists working in the Disability Resource Centre, and 'helpers'. The latter are basically students who do not have physical impairments, and whose major task is to assist physically challenged students with special tasks such as laundry, writing assignments, and the use of technical equipment such as computers. On the other hand, we have students who are physically challenged. The former group is the 'oppressor' category, while the latter is the oppressed group. In this project, using action-research typology, both groups are involved in self-learning and self-discovery. As a result, it could be argued that all of the relevant stakeholders are involved in genuine and democratic dialogue that is critical in solving human problems associated

---

[2] John Gaventa & Andrea Cornwall, "Power and Knowledge," in *A Handbook of Action Research*, ed. Peter Reason & Hilary Bradbury (Thousand Oaks CA & London: Sage, 2006): 174.

[3] Patricia Maguire, "Uneven Ground: Feminisms and Action Research," in *A Handbook of Action Research*, ed. Peter Reason & Hilary Bradbury (Thousand Oaks CA & London: Sage, 2006): 60–70.

[4] Gaventa & Cornwall, "Power and Knowledge," 179.

[5] Jean McNiff & Jack Whitehead, *Action Research for Teachers: A Practical Guide* (London: David Fulton, 2005): 1.

[6] McNiff & Whitehead, *Action Research for Teachers: A Practical Guide*, 1.

with development in its broad sense. This is consistent with the following observation:

> Action research is a participatory, democratic process concerned with developing practical knowing in the pursuit of worthwhile human purposes grounded in a participatory world-view we believe is emerging at this historical moment. It seeks to bring together action and reflecting theory and practice in participation with others, in the practical solutions to issues of practical concern to the people, and more generally the nourishing of individual persons and their community.[7]

A typical example of the democratic nature of the project is that all so-called able-bodied persons necessarily concede that they belong to the 'oppressor' group in a broad sense. Comments and references to this fact are made in non-threatening, humorous, but serious tones and contexts. These are some of the practical processes that are made in "the pursuit of the worthwhile human purposes" that are referred to in the above quotation.

In the light of the above, one of the key features of action research which should make it 'attractive' to TfD ideals and practices is that it is a relational knowledge which is "the foundation of community life and its development fosters community ties as well as helping to create other forms of knowledge."[8] Relationships are therefore very critical to the success of action research. This project seeks to animate students with physical impairments to realize that they can construct their own knowledge which directly affects their lived experiences and produces practical knowledge of immediate use. Even in an apparently technical context such as HIV/AIDS, it is of central importance in action-research typology to treat participants or project beneficiaries as "competent cognizers"[9] whose knowledge is essential to the pursuit of solutions to challenges affecting them.

In short, there are many possibilities that can be realized by the application of the principles and techniques of action research. One of the chief potential outcomes is the creation of democratic processes of interaction or engagement as an ideal forum for articulating and expressing ideas which can lead to practical action in alleviating even sensitive social and emotional issues affecting disempowered groups in their lived experiences. However, there are also

---

[7] Peter Reason & Hilary Bradbury, ed. *A Handbook of Action Research* (Thousand Oaks CA & London: Sage, 2006): 1.

[8] Reason & Bradbury, ed. *A Handbook of Action Research*, 10.

[9] McNiff & Whitehead, *Action Research for Teachers: A Practical Guide*.

many challenges and tensions which can be encountered in an attempt to apply the principles of action research in TfD practice and, in this case, HIV/AIDS related TfD practice. Subsequent sections will cite some typical examples of such challenges and tensions – particularly those relating to a multidisciplinary approach to HIV/AIDS communication in TfD practice.

Theorization

Disability is constructed here as a social problem using the Social Model, where disability is a disadvantage or restriction of activity caused by a contemporary social organization which takes no or little account of people whose physical impairments exclude them from participating in the mainstream of social actions.[10] The Social Model of disability does not deny the reality of physical impairments, but it focuses on the failure of society and social systems to provide relevant and appropriate facilities and services in order to ameliorate social and economic situations that affect these groups of people.[11] In this project, therefore, the main focus is to examine analytical and aesthetic tools that can be used to critically challenge ideologies and prejudices that perpetuate discrimination and marginalization of people living with physical impairments. Consequently, elements of empowerment which are critical for this project include (a) organization of affected people, (b) social awareness, (c) self-reliance, (d) development of creative capacities, and (e) solidarity.[12]

Two major observations inform theoretical approaches to this study. In the first instance, it is evident that while indeed modernization theories have generally been contested in principle in Africa, in practice they continue to influence TfD projects and processes. For example, it is usually argued that modernization theory is too technical, consumeristic, and 'foreign' to socio-political systems in Africa.[13] However, in Zimbabwe, for an example, most

---

[10] Michael Oliver, *The Politics of Disablement* (Basingstoke & London: Macmillan Education, 1990).

[11] Oliver, *The Politics of Disablement.*

[12] M. Anisur Rahman, *People's Self-Development: Perspectives on Participatory Action Research; a journey through experience* (London & Atlantic Highlands NJ: Zed; Dhaka: Dhaka UP, 1993): 202.

[13] John Mukim Mbaku, *Institutions and Development in Africa* (Trenton NJ: Africa World Press, 2004).

projects can be criticized on the basis that they copy 'Western' notions of development that emphasize technology, capital, and consumerism.

If this criticism is to be applied to HIV/AIDS interventions in the context of disability, it can be argued that care should be taken to avoid too much emphasis on condom use, provision of drugs, food for affected patients, and other 'technologies' related to human sexuality at the expense of critical engagement with social processes which marginalize and disempower oppressed groups. In this regard, the major motivation is to pursue holistic, relational, cultural, and ideological forms of empowerment in HIV/AIDS theatrical interventions.

The second observation is that theorization of development relevant to Africa has moved almost exclusively in the Marxist orbit.[14] However, it is very important to consider multidisciplinary approaches that take into account not only local realities but also other adaptable foreign paradigms. Consequently, major theories that inform the study include participatory democratic theory, public choice theory, the Freirean theory of conscientization, experiential-learning theory, the poetics of the oppressed, social-learning theory, and feminist theory.

The above theories and paradigms emphasize qualitative analytical tools which pursue democracy, liberation, and empowerment. They all acknowledge that social realities emanate from social constructions which can be challenged and modified to ameliorate human suffering. They are grounded in a socio-political approach which explores qualitative dimensions of development such as love, emotional maturity, and development of creative capacities, human rights, and freedom. Directly or indirectly, these theories seek to instil among oppressed groups the desire to change oppressive systems.

It is submitted here that the complexity of oppression in the arena of disability requires that one consider multidisciplinary approaches in order to derive maximum benefit from many theoretical considerations. This is necessary in order to unravel and challenge the multiple layers of oppression characterizing this apparently much neglected area of human existence.

However, there are some challenges that arise from the infusion and merging of such diverse approaches in one project. The first obvious challenge is that a research study which deploys many diverse paradigms can easily lose

---

[14] Hyden Goran, "Changing Ideological and Theoretical Perspectives on Development," in *African Perspectives on Development*, ed. Ulf Himmerlstrand, Kabiru Kinyanjiui & E.K. Mburugu (New York: James Currey, 1994): 308–19.

focus and depth. There are inevitable tensions that arise from working with social scientists from diverse fields. For example, some social scientists and practitioners in this project have questioned the 'objectivity' of participatory approaches. On the other hand, HIV/AIDS specialists are keen on giving scientific 'truth' and information and not subjecting these 'scientific' processes to critical examination. Yet, ideally in TfD practice, nothing should be sacrosanct. During one of the workshops to construct storylines for this project, there was an interesting discussion which can serve to illustrate the tension under discussion. A theatre-arts student suggested that the source of most myths surrounding the sexuality of people living with physical impairments would be the church. A social scientist challenged this suggestion on the basis that it was unrealistic and offensive. Here was a typical example of the tension between artistic truth/possibilities and scientific 'objectivity'. In fact, when working with social scientists in a TfD project, it is always important to be alert to the reality that they can suspect or insinuate that artists cannot be very useful in addressing 'serious scientific' realities. For example, it has been suggested that theatre is not so subject to empiricism as sociology, psychology, and economics.[15] This is to assert that theatre is non-empirical. This perspective probably emanates from the exaggeration of the recognition that theatre as an artform enjoys poetic licence. Harmonizing this poetic licence with some social science 'objective' paradigms can be a real challenge.

Notwithstanding the above, I contend that an interdisciplinary approach to TfD theorization can provide profound insights into the realities of disempowered social groups and possible means to empowering and liberating them. For example, applying the main principles of direct participatory democratic theory has ensured that all participants with physical impairments can articulate their social, aesthetic, and emotional concerns with limited inhibitions. At the same time, considerations of feminist theorists have been critical in ensuring that gender oppressions are not overlooked in a quest to challenge discrimination based on disability. Consequently, it has become relatively easier to problematize rather than 'preach' social problems relating to HIV/AIDS and disability. In addition, the Social Model that is being deployed to interrogate disability in a way that is liberatory is based on theorization on disability from sociological perspectives. Lastly, action-research practices are

---

[15] Justus Mwanje, "The Qualitative and Quantitative Social Science Research Processes" (unpublished paper presented at the Methodological Workshop for Social Science Research in Africa, Nairobi, 10–14 August 2009).

inspired by experiential-learning theory, which postulates that effective and transformational learning comes from combining cognitive and affective domains. Experiential learning is "a four-stage cycle involving four learning modes; concrete experience, reflective observation, abstract conceptualism and active experimentation."[16] Drama workshops, rehearsals, and improvisations are vehicles through which the above ideals are applied to provide a reflective and transformational learning experience for students who face various forms of discrimination as a result of their physical disabilities.

The point here is that considerations of diverse theoretical paradigms tend to deepen and enrich the understanding of social factors relating to participatory TfD practices.

In any case, the differences between theatre and the social sciences have been unnecessarily exaggerated. Theatre is a multi-media discipline which relates to many disciplines such as literature, history, religion, politics, education, and sociology. For example, in trying to emphasize this point, Jonothan Needlands has submitted that theatre is "active sociology."[17] I further submit that applied theatre relates much more to the social science domain than do any other sub-categories of theatre. Before discussing some of the specific possibilities that can be realized from such an approach, the next section discusses ethical challenges in a project of such a nature.

Situated Ethical Issues

In research involving oppressed groups, one is always faced with serious ethical tensions and dilemmas. In this research, these ethical considerations are further complicated by the sensitivity of the topic being dealt with. The usual challenge of the autonomy of participants to make informed consent in participation was not serious in this project, since participants are educated people with an appreciation of the requirements of research processes. At the beginning, the participants clearly expressed their suspicions about, and reluctance to participate in, the project, based on their previous experiences with other researchers. It took some months of persuasion and negotiation to convince them to participate. And in each phase of the project we always

[16] David A. Kolb, *Experiential Learning: Experience as the Source of Learning and Development* (Englewood Cliffs NJ: Prentice–Hall, 1984): 16.

[17] Jonothan Neelands, *Making Sense of Drama: A Guide to Classroom Practice* (1984; Oxford: Heinemann Educational, 1989).

reviewed the partnership and modified the 'contract' in accordance with changing circumstances. However, one of the questions we have been discussing as animators is that of providing refreshments in all our meetings. In ordinary circumstances, this cannot be an issue. Yet it must be noted that ethical issues are contextual.[18] Thus, in 2007 and 2008 in Zimbabwe, provision of refreshments which were extremely scant could be interpreted as inducements, which can be considered to be unethical.

There is also tension between the need to maintain confidentiality and the ideal in action research to solve immediate practical problems affecting participants. Action research does not work with abstract concepts but deals with real-life practical situations affecting communities. Now, when dealing with sensitive issues such as HIV/AIDS and sexuality, it is not easy to be specific about one's experiences. In any case, theatre is not so much a private space as a public arena. For example, we used the workshop technique to create storylines. This was done collectively. However, at the start, participants had inhibitions which made it difficult for them to express themselves freely on emotional and sexual issues, so the workshop method was not sufficient to solicit personal observations on sensitive issues from them. Personal experiences and observations are critical in action research in order to tackle real issues. There is need for private interviews and any other means where sensitive issues can be revealed without exposing the identity of an informant. For example, it was easy for 'oppressors' to reveal emotional and personal observations and experiences on sexuality during a workshop. However, it was not easy for some female 'helpers' to express their concerns about what they considered to be unethical conduct from some young men with physical impairments, who, it is alleged, asked for sexual favours from 'able-bodied' female 'helpers'. Apparently, this was overstretching the functions of 'helpers'. In the first instance, this is a complication of the oppressor–oppressed dynamic. The fundamental question here, however, is: How do you deal with such sensitive issues, which are real, because, in the project, one of the guiding principles is the need for robust and democratic interaction? But to what extent can such issues be discussed without hurting the feelings of the 'disempowered'? Navigating such situated ethical issues can be very precarious. It

---

[18] Barbara Thomas–Slayter, "A brief history of participatory methodologies," in *Power Process and Participation: Tools for Change*, ed. Rachel Slocum, Lori Wichhart, Dianne Rocheleau & Barbara Thomas–Slayter (London: Intermediate Technology, 1995): 10–17.

requires tact, sensitivity, diplomacy, good public relations, and intellectual acumen.

Another ethical challenge was realized at the level of creating scenes, which in this project proved to be very effective in dismantling pervasive myths about the sexuality of people living with physical impairments. However, in an effort to maintain the spirit of inclusivity and equality, the scenes created raised certain expectations of romantic relationships between people with physical impairments and those without. Yet, in reality, there could still remain some prejudice and discrimination. The question is: Should fictional scenarios raise expectations that cannot be immediately realized by a disempowered group? In addition, it is difficult to anticipate the level of emotional sensitivity of marginalized participants. In the workshop referred to above, there were scenic paraphernalia which formed the basis for the construction of storylines for the performance. Some of the items present were torn or disfigured condoms. A visually impaired young lady was given one of the condoms to have a 'feel', and she was visibly disturbed at being made to touch a condom. It is not clear why she was so disturbed. This only goes to show that situated ethics can be extremely difficult to apply. It takes a great deal of experience, sensitivity, and relational competence to contain and forestall situations which can potentially provoke sensitive emotions.

Lastly, the ethical principle of beneficence requires that the research be of social benefit, even though the subjects themselves may not benefit directly from participating.[19] To an extent, this project has already yielded some positive benefits, some of which do apply directly to participants. For example, one art-and-design student has been challenged by the scenes which show that physically impaired people are disadvantaged when it comes to HIV/AIDS information and she has designed posters in braille for the benefit of the visually impaired, posters which were displayed on 10 November 2009 at an art exhibition. In addition, last year's performance depicted the insensitivity of lecturers who do not normally consider the needs of people with physical impairments in their delivery of lectures. In response to this revelation, a vigorous campaign has been launched to alert lecturers to be sensitive to the needs of physically challenged students. Yet a dilemma arises when disempowered participants expect more 'tangible' benefits. For example, some actors wanted

---

[19] Mary van der Riet, Angela Hough & Bev Killian, "Mapping HIV/AIDS as a Barrier to Education: A Reflection on Methodological and Ethical Challenges to Child Participation," *Journal of Education* 35 (2005): 75–98.

allowances for rehearsals. If such expectations are fulfilled, to what extent would we say we have not induced or coerced participation?

In a nutshell, while situated ethics are challenging in implementation, they can be navigated by being sensitive and alert to the social dynamics of a given context.

Animation – Facilitation Dialectics

In development theory, there is a difference between animation and facilitation. Generally, animation refers to thought-based processes which break down mental barriers to self-liberation. It is based on the Freiriean theory of conscientization – of self-reflected awareness on the part of oppressed people of their social reality, revealing their ability to transform it by their conscious action.[20] Facilitation, by contrast, refers to the practical aspects of breaking down practical barriers to action. Examples of such actions could include the acquisition of basic skills such as literacy and supply of information about legislation and policies.[21] The challenge that has been encountered in this project, especially when dealing with many partners, is: Which of the two should take priority? Generally, it would be ideal if participatory TfD were to concentrate mainly on animation in order to emphasize psychological, intellectual, and ideological empowerment. In an endeavour to emphasize this aspect, character-construction was motivated by the desire to avoid treating people with disabilities as passive and pitiable, or as 'victims' of impairment. The idea was to construct characters with strengths and weaknesses facing socially constructed barriers which can be challenged. This year, for instance, the main protagonist is a visually impaired young woman who is both a 'heroine' and a 'villain' at the same time.

However, communities who have been subjected to marginalization, disempowerment, and abuse for a long time tend to want facilitation more than animation. For example, in this project, there has been much enthusiasm about technical issues such as the proper use of a condom. There is nothing wrong with imparting relevant technical and practical information and skills. However, there is danger that participatory TfD projects can degenerate into HIV/AIDS 'propaganda' or, in this case, 'condom propaganda'. This would not be consistent with conscientization, which thrives on problematization. To

---

[20] Rahman, *People's Self-Development*, 81.

[21] *People's Self-Development*, 81.

this extent, it becomes highly imperative that applied-theatre practitioners work in close partnership with social-science theorists and practitioners in a multidisciplinary context. This will make it possible for HIV/AIDS technical experts to concentrate on facilitation, while applied-theatre theorist–practitioners focus on animation, because it is the creative aspects, including dramatic parody, humour, conflict, sarcasm, spectacle, witticism, and subtext, that can stimulate critical engagement with social phenomenon. In short, this project is inspired by the recognition that facilitation should be subordinate to animation.[22]

Socio-Relational Dynamics

It has already been noted that qualitative dimensions of development emphasize human dignity, self-esteem, self-actualization, human freedom, and human rights.[23] These are based on democratic principles and ideals. To this extent, it became very evident, in the project under discussion, that the success of TfD methodology, especially when using action-research instruments, requires open, genuine, and beneficial social interaction with project beneficiaries or participants.

In pursuit of this ideal, a number of practical steps were undertaken. Informal meetings outside the project context were arranged. These included social visits to the residence of project beneficiaries and attending social functions, such as parties, together with people with physical impairments. Animators and research participants shared social messages on cell phones and emails. In social discussions, inside or outside of a formal setting, it is critical to acknowledge the full humanity of people with disabilities, including their strengths and human weaknesses. It is in this regard critical to share non-offensive humour and jokes. Differences are discussed and acknowledged in a non-threatening environment.

We can draw parallels with achievement-motivation theory, which contends that students can be easily motivated if they perceive that what they are learning is personally meaningful and relevant and when they are in sup-

---

[22] Peter Du Sautoy, *The Organisation of a Community Development Programme* (Oxford: Oxford UP, 1962).

[23] Charles Chachage, "The Discourse on Development Among African Philosophers," in *African Perspectives on Development*, ed. Ulf Himmerlstrand, Kabiru Kinyanjiui & E.K. Mburugu (New York: James Currey, 1994): 51–73.

portive interactions with their teachers. This is crucial to enhancing self-esteem.[24]

In this regard, it is of paramount importance in action research to employ practical social instruments to create social engagements that enhance democracy, freedom, cooperation, trust, and confidence. This can psychologically empower marginalized groups to be able to discuss sensitive issues with minimum inhibition. For example, a number of scenes were conceived and created by physically challenged participants which explored their psychic concerns and aspirations about human sexuality and HIV/AIDS. As a result of positive social engagement, it became very easy for students with physical challenges to volunteer in all the creative aspects of the project. Some worked on developing scenes at rehearsals, others on acting and directing. Another interesting dimension to the creative process is that two physically challenged participants volunteered to become jokers at a performance workshop held in January 2010, in which representatives of all university stakeholders participated. There are many creative possibilities for people with physical challenges if they are sufficiently animated, motivated, and trained. In this regard, I contend here that the highest ideals and aspirations of creative and intellectual participation of affected and disempowered groups are only achievable in an environment where social interactions between them and animators are at their highest peak in terms of mutual trust and sincerity. This can be realized, provided that animators are sufficiently equipped with relational competence.

Conclusion

This article has explored the relationship between action research and TfD research methodology. There are close links between the two, suggesting that research methodology in TfD practice is to some extent action research. One of the key observations has been that action research and TfD practice share the same theoretical inspirations. However, there are some principles, techniques, and practices in action research that could be extremely useful if they are explicitly and systematically applied in TfD practices, particularly those projects dealing with marginalized communities who suffer from complex and multiple forms of oppression. In the project under discussion, appropriation of these action-research principles and practices has witnessed both

[24] Barbara L. McCombs & James E. Pope, *Developing Essential Study Skills* (Essex: Pearson Education, 1994).

challenges and immense social, ideological, psychological, and creative empowerment possibilities. It is submitted here that these possibilities can be actualized in a context where, methodologically and theoretically, multi-disciplinary theoretical perspectives which privilege human integrity, sense of community, democracy, human rights, and human dignity are applied consistently and systematically. I contend that these analytical frameworks and methodological practices work effectively if animators are sufficiently equipped with relational competence, a critical requirement when dealing with disempowered communities. In conclusion, I suggest that such a multi-disciplinary approach can animate physically challenged people to challenge and change social barriers which disadvantage them in HIV/AIDS discourses and practices.

WORKS CITED

Chachage, Charles. "The Discourse on Development Among African Philosophers," in *African Perspectives on Development*, ed. Ulf Himmerlstrand, Kabiru Kinyanjiui & E.K. Mburugu (New York: James Currey, 1994): 51–73.

Du Sautoy, Peter. *The Organisation of a Community Development Programme* (Oxford: Oxford UP, 1962).

Gaventa, John, & Andrea Cornwall. "Power and Knowledge," in *A Handbook of Action Research*, ed. Peter Reason & Hilary Bradbury (Thousand Oaks CA & London: Sage, 2006): 172–89.

Goran, Hyden. "Changing Ideological and Theoretical Perspectives on Development," in *African Perspectives on Development*, ed. Ulf Himmerlstrand, Kabiru Kinyanjiui & E.K. Mburugu (New York: James Currey, 1994): 308–19.

Kolb, David A. *Experiential Learning: Experience as the Source of Learning and Development* (Englewood Cliffs NJ: Prentice–Hall, 1984).

Maguire, Patricia. "Uneven Ground: Feminisms and Action Research," in *A Handbook of Action Research*, ed. Peter Reason & Hilary Bradbury (Thousand Oaks CA & London: Sage, 2006): 60–70.

Mbaku, John Mukim. *Institutions and Development in Africa* (Trenton NJ: Africa World Press, 2004).

McCombs, Barbara L., & James E. Pope. *Developing Essential Study Skills* (Essex: Pearson Education, 1994).

McNiff, Jean, & Jack Whitehead. *Action Research for Teachers: A Practical Guide* (London: David Fulton, 2005).

Mwanje, Justus. "The Qualitative and Quantitative Social Science Research Processes" (unpublished paper presented at the Methodological Workshop for Social Science Research in Africa. Nairobi 10–14 August 2009).

Neelands, Jonothan. *Making Sense of Drama: A Guide to Classroom Practice* (1984; Oxford: Heinemann Educational, 1989).

Oliver, Michael. *The Politics of Disablement* (Basingstoke & London: Macmillan Education, 1990).

Rahman, M. Anisur. *People's Self-Development: Perspectives on Participatory Action Research; a journey through experience* (London & Atlantic Highlands NJ: Zed; Dhaka: Dhaka UP, 1993).

Reason, Peter, & Hilary Bradbury, ed. *A Handbook of Action Research* (Thousand Oaks CA & London: Sage, 2006).

Thomas–Slayter, Barbara. "A brief history of participatory methodologies," in *Power Process and Participation: Tools for Change*, ed. Rachel Slocum, Lori Wichhart, Dianne Rocheleau & Barbara Thomas–Slayter (London: Intermediate Technology, 1995): 10–17.

Van der Riet, Mary, Angela Hough & Bev Killian. "Mapping HIV/AIDS as a Barrier to Education: A Reflection on Methodological and Ethical Challenges to Child Participation," *Journal of Education* 35 (2005): 75–98.

⌘

INNOVATIONS IN HIV/AIDS AWARENESS EDUCATION

DIANA WILSON AND KAREN SUTER

The Lover and Another

A Consideration of the Efficacy of Utilizing a Performance Poetry Competition as Vehicle for HIV/AIDS Education Among Young Adults

THIS ESSAY CONCERNS 'The Lover and Another', a performance-poetry competition devised and run by Diana Wilson and Karen Suter, members of the Drama and Performance Studies staff at the University of KwaZulu–Natal, Pietermaritzburg during the second semester of 2009. This initiative was a response to a call from Applied Arts for HIV/AIDS Awareness (AAA-HA!) and funded by DramAidE to find innovative ways of using the performing arts to raise student awareness of the dangers of multiple partnerships in the context of the high HIV/AIDS infection rates in this age group. We suggest that the writing and performance of a single poem within the structure of a competition run over several rounds may enable a participant to produce communication of sufficient aesthetic quality to engage effectively with an audience. The essay will first consider a single poem in the competition before giving the rationale of using performance poetry for HIV/ AIDS education. This will be followed by an outline of how the competition was structured and implemented before considering whether, how, and why this type of intervention might be useful both to an audience and to the participants themselves in creating an openness about HIV/AIDS-related issues. Any insights are based on information gathered from audience and participant surveys conducted with questionnaires devised by AAA-HA!, in-depth interviews with three of the participating poets several weeks after the competition, and the organizers' observations of the processes engaged in by the participants.

The following poem was written and performed by a first-year student, Joy Dlamini, in the final of this competition before an audience of over three hundred young men and women. In addition to the text, some notes about the audience reaction audible on the recording of the performance have been added.

SUGAR DADDY [*audience echoes 'Sugar Daddy'*]

I don't care if I'm about to date a man old enough to be my father
I don't give a damn if I'm about to destroy the marriage
of a woman old enough to be my own mother
I don't care if he has got another lover or multiple partners
Yah abanye bayagwayabangibiza ngamagama
but if udaddy ephaka ngeke ngikwazi ukumgaba [*audience: whoops, yells 'Sshhh!'*]

Buy me a phone and I'll give you access
to all my assets
Pay me well we won't need to wrestle

You see different men approach me on a daily basis
They hide their rings so that I can satisfy their needs
without my conscience bugging me

You call me names and say I've got no conscience
But try being me for a day
Maybe then you'll understand
that it's hard to be jobless and penniless
Knowing you walk around with this illness
just makes it worse
I am cursed
and tired of defending myself

You see, as a child daddy came to my room every night
He said open wide daddy only want to touch
But that touch led to a suck
A suck followed by a painful, painful penetration *audience: aaah !ah! sshh...*]
See daddy prepared me for this business
He taught me the different positions
That's how I got my qualifications [*audience: huge reaction: 'Whooo hah!'*]

Yeah, a once innocent virgin,
now surrounded by walls of HIV
depending on ARVs to survive
Yet I continue to pass this virus on to these multiple partners
Who pass it on to their wives.
Yes I continue taking innocent lives

You talk about love
I don't have love for I've never been loved
All I have is the seeds of this greed
That grow inside me,
They cause me to bleed

I scream and I weep
as I try to ignore
This disease I am fighting.
Yes, I weep even more
as I try to ignore this disease I am fighting
facing
I am at war
Yes we are at war. [*audience: erupts in applause*]

It is important to note that there was no directorial intervention of any kind in the creation of the performance. It is all Joy Dlamini's own work; she wrote the poem and decided how she would present it to the audience. In the context of this conference, a key question is perhaps whether this unmediated creative work by participants has the capacity for effective communication with an audience. In other words, does the vehicle of a student performance-poetry competition allow for sufficient aesthetic quality to achieve effective communication around the complexities of HIV/AIDS? The audience response heard on this recording indicates that it does, but it might be worthwhile to consider whether the process of writing and performing a poem within the structure of the competition may in itself have contributed to the development of the participant's performance skills. To begin to answer this question, the rationale of using performance poetry should first be explained.

At the time of conceptualizing this project there was an apparent student interest in performance poetry on the Pietermaritzburg campus of KwaZulu–Natal. For instance, asked to select a poem to work on in a drama tutorial, students would often choose rap poems; there were groups in student residences who met to perform their poems; and there were several articles in the local press about performance-poetry competitions. We felt that this interest could possibly be harnessed to engage an audience's interest and create a platform for students to express their own ideas and hopes and feelings about their lives and relationships. We considered that this could possibly be more interesting for both audiences and participants alike than devising and staging a play with a predetermined message. Consequently, a decision was made to offer prize money which might lure participants into entering the competition, the rules of which would then require them to focus on theme of the dangers of multiple partners.

It might be worthwhile to consider briefly what contributes to the popularity of performance poetry that we were proposing to exploit. We would suggest that there are several factors involved. One is that audiences respond to the skill with which the performers manipulate language: there is admiration for the poet's use of alliteration, assonance, rhythm, and wit. Secondly, the musicality of the spoken language is delightful in itself and often heightens deeply felt emotions in the audience. Lastly, within the confines of a single poem there is also scope for dramatic narrative and characterization that is appealing to audiences. If, to these factors, are added the competitive element and the challenge of focusing the poems on the potentially taboo area of private sexuality, then there is excitement about the competition itself and audience admiration for the courage of the participants.

The social and political engagement with the subject-matter of much performance poetry is often apparent. Cornelia Gräbner suggests that the presence of the poet at the site of performance in a public space emphasizes his or her membership of the community and this is further reinforced by the use of the "vernaculars, dialects and accents. Usually speech that is marked by any of the three situates the poet within a particular community."[1] She uses the terms "sonic layering" and "layers of signification" for the use of "music, rhythm, recordings or imitations of nonverbal sounds [...] oftentimes performed simultaneously with other elements of signification" (5) which are characteristic of performance poetry. In terms of this initiative, it was important that there was the opportunity for participants to develop a layered communication with members of their own communication about the implications of living at a time of HIV infection rates.

---

[1] Cornelia Gräbner, "Performance Poetry: New Languages and New Literary Circuits?," *World Literature Today* 82.1 (January–February 2008): 21 paras, http://eprints .lancs .ac.uk/14200/1/Poetics_of_Performance_Poetry.pdf (accessed 13 January 2010), para 4.

The competition was structured to run over the first five weeks of the second semester. The first week was devoted to publicity for the launch event, which was scheduled in the second week. The publicity consisted of bright yellow-and-blue posters with the prize money prominently displayed. These posters informed the reader that the subject-matter of the poems was to be about "the complexities of relationships" that any type of poetry was allowed, not just slam and rap, and the dates, times, and venues of the launch event and the 'Mega Final' which was to be held in the Students' Union. In addition, to give more information about thelaunch event and the audition rounds, fliers were distributed with more than a hundred free bright-yellow bow-ties, made by a team of volunteer drama students. These bow-ties were very popular and worn almost everywhere except round the neck. Their bright visibility enabled us to see how the message about the competition was spreading around the campus. In addition to the posters and fliers, information was also available on the drama-studies website.

The free launch event was important for several reasons: we wanted to encourage participants to enter the competition; we needed to give an idea of the variety of performance styles that could be used; we wanted to create a 'buzz' of excitement about the competition and to assess whether there was indeed any student interest in the project. The venue for this launch and the subsequent audition rounds and semi-final was the foyer to the Hexagon Theatre, adjacent to the popular coffee bar, where there is a high volume of student traffic. This foyer space is already equipped with a small platform stage, and a microphone and sound system were supplied for the events by the Hexagon Theatre. Initially, students simply brought in chairs from the coffee bar if they wanted to sit, but this rapidly became incorporated into the regular set-up. All the events were held late mornings or lunchtimes during the week so students were already on campus, and, because we wanted to create visibility for the competition in the hope of attracting passers-by and those students who would not usually attend a performance in a theatre, there was a banner above the entrance, music was played over the sound system, and the venue was decorated both outside and inside with the blue-and-yellow balloons, which became the visual signal that events in the competition were taking place.

At the launch event, after performances of poetry of various styles in both English and isiZulu by invited performers from within the drama department and several slam poems by Nkululeko Mdlala, a guest poet from Platform Poets, the rules were explained and sign-up sheets and entry forms were made available. These entry forms had attached to them the rules of the competition and the handout 'Relationships and More' devised for us by Emma Durden of AAA-HA! (see Appendix 2) The sign-up sheets requested the cell-phone number of the participant concerned and thereafter all communication about progress through the competition was made to participants by sms and to audience members through notices in the Hexagon Theatre foyer space. Judging for the three audition rounds and the semifinal was done anonymously by Ntokozo Madlala, lecturer in Drama and Performance Studies, and Arifani Moyo, a recent Drama Masters student, using the criteria set out in the rules:

> 10. Contestants will be judged on their performance and the originality, creativity and effectiveness of their communication of the ideas set out in the "Relationships and more..." guidelines to this competition.

Of the thirty-five students who entered the competition, there were an almost equal numbers of men and women, registered for subjects such as law, business studies, sociology, economics, drama, and media, and they were in their first to fourth year of study. Through the process of elimination, the number was reduced to twenty-one in the semi-final and to fifteen in the final. Audience numbers for the preliminary rounds ranged from seventy to 120.

To attract a larger audience, the change of venue to the much bigger Students' Union, booked for the final, required greater publicity efforts. As an added attraction, we devised a lucky draw for the audience with prizes solicited from local businesses patronized largely by students. In addition to articles in the press, on the day of the event several drama students doing a technical-management course painted themselves blue and urged fellow students into the Hall. As audience members went in they were given numbered handouts of the 'Relationships and More' handout, which then became the tickets for the lucky draw. The venue was decorated with the competition's signature blue-and-yellow balloons; photos of the finalists and all the poems entered in the competition were displayed. There were three external judges for the final: Emma Durden from AAA-HA!, Brian Khoza, a local poet and journalist, and the poet Nqobile Ntsangase. The finalists drew for performance order and performed their poems interspersed with audience draws for prizes. After the judges' deliberations, the winners were announced.

The growing audience numbers and large, excited audience at the final demonstrated that it was a very popular competition, but we need to question whether this initiative was effective in achieving its aims in terms of HIV/AIDS education. Perhaps some idea of the multi-facetted and rich communication that the audience attending the final received about issues relating to the complexities of lives lived in the context of high HIV infection rates may be gained from a summary of the subject-matter of the poems presented at this event: (Some information regarding performance style is included where relevant.)

— Questioning the nature of love itself (*dialogue between speaker with old man, humorously vocally characterized*);
— our eternal pursuit of money (*chorus, picked up and chanted back by audience*);
— poet questions why a girl would kill her young husband who has loved her loyally since being fellow students by giving him HIV caught from an older rich man with whom she'd had a relationship while at university;
— a kiss, which leads the speaker into marriage with a polygamist;
— the prohibitions placed on women's behaviour by male strictures:
  - a successful businesswoman's confession that she has been having an affair and lying about her love for her husband (*guitar accompaniment and a sung chorus*);
  - the anguish of a young mother who cannot question her husband about her realization that the woman she saw at his funeral was the 'other' who has given her the virus;
  - a plea to young women not to be used by men 'like small house' but to live the life they deserve;
  - the HI virus as the unwelcome visitor in the speaker's body (*with guitar accompaniment*);
  - a young man's feelings of powerless anger as he sees his sister selling her favours to an older man;
  - a plea by a person with HIV to not give him sentimental sympathy until the listener has 'cried his tears';
  - a song of cynical seduction and abandonment 'the morning after' (*up-beat rap with pre-recorded backing track*);
  - a decision to remain abstinent until marriage to avoid the contradictions surrounding love;
— the loneliness which leads the speaker to take a ride in a 'lust-mobile';
— the poet's love of rap being his first love – his girlfriend being 'the other'.

It would be difficult for a scripted play to contain such a variety of content, but the question remains as to whether the participants had sufficient performance skill to communicate these often complex ideas to an audience. The observed audience reaction and audience surveys suggest strongly that this was so, and the interviews with three of the finalists were particularly revealing about how the task of performing a poem within the structure of the competition in itself contributed to a growing concern with the aesthetic aspects of their performances. Four factors were identified: the competitive nature of a competition (as the word suggests); the urge to communicate a message thought to be important; the challenge of the required focus; and, perhaps most importantly, the interactive nature of the communication between poets and audiences.

The three interviewees said that they were motivated to enter the competition not only by the prize money but also because they enjoyed writing and performing poetry and thought they could test themselves against others and develop their skills. There was rivalry among participants to present the best work, but this, they said, was not aggressive. All remarked on the friendly atmosphere in which the competition was run and commented generously on the quality of other participants' performances. Two of the three asserted that although their initial motivation might have been to win a competition, once they engaged with gathering information and their own thoughts and feelings in order to fulfil the task of writing a poem focused on the complexity of the issues surrounding HIV/AIDS, they felt a growing need to be courageous and frank in their urge to alert their peers to the real dangers they perceived. All said that the 'Relationships and More' handout was seminal to this process, guiding them to write in a more personal, emotional style and to consider the required subject-matter from a more complex, less fact-driven perspective. One interviewee said: "I used to write da da dah Christian poems and then I read that 'Relationships and More' and realized I could write about myself, my experiences and what I feel." They found seeing how other poets approached the same subject-matter interesting, challenging, and often eye-opening. For instance, another interviewee said about the rap-song poem 'The Morning After': "We were singing along, joining in the chorus, and then realized this guy was breaking some sort of male code letting girls know that men behave like this."

They all commented on the challenge of speaking about sexuality in public, that it was difficult. One remarked that she was glad her mother had not seen the performance, and another that she had had to explain to a member of her church group that she was adopting a persona when she was accused of being 'raunchy'. The third explained that performing a poem in public is different from public speaking because it has a rhythm that 'carries you along'.

In addition, they all said that the structure of the competition to run over several rounds helped them assess audience reaction and adapt and develop their poems and their performances so that they could communicate more effectively. For instance, after the first round, one poet brought in her guitar and turned the poem into a song, which added another rich layer to her performance. All three interviewees stressed that the dynamic nature of the performer/audience relationship was crucial to the way they honed their work. One said, "When you get to the end of your poem, and there's an mmmmm and then silence.... and then cheers and applause – you know they understand you."

Further, all three remarked that being part of the competition has had an impact on their lives. The public platform of the competition has meant that they have become recognized figures on campus, and are often greeted in a friendly way with quotations from their competition poems. All three said that both men and women still, several months after 'The Lover and Another' initiative, stop and want to talk to them about their poems and the ideas they expressed. However, the impact of the competition has perhaps been felt most by Nokwethemba Mchunu, whose winning poem is printed below. It was clear from her first audition round that she managed to generate an extraordinary audience reaction and people were very excited by her performance and clearly identified with her message. This poem has become so popular that she has been invited to perform it at church groups, at women's groups, at AIDS awareness gatherings both on campus and in the wider community, but also, more surprisingly perhaps, at the Ball for the Petrie residence and the Ball for the Humanities students. This suggests very strongly that a performance-poetry competition can be an entertaining and popular way of generating an openness and discussion around HIV/AIDS-related issues among university students.

Contradictions

Once upon a time we believed in happily ever after
but relationships it seems we have not, cannot and will never master
See now, LOVE, LOVE, LOVE to most does not exist
But LUST it seems we cannot resist
it persists so persistent, never consistent, due to the existence

of predictable, predicted, predictions of contradictions, contradicting this thing called LOVE

Boys with their mouths LOVE they confess
But deep down we know it's all about the sex
with, NO without condom protection for their pathetic perception is that
"Girl your love for me without skin on skin sex
means you are at risk of being my ex"
And because Love for herself she lacked
she gave him that which she could never take back
her virgin innocence was licence assurance to him that she did in fact sincerely love him
The existence of predictable, predicted, predictions of contradictions that contradict this thing called LOVE

The words I LOVE YOU are always spoken
but somehow you always leave me broken
It seems that our love will forever stand as you caress, care, comfort me when I'm sad, mad
but yet you beat bat abuse me with that very same hand
the existence of predictable predicted predictions of contradictions that contradict this thing called LOVE

Verbally you love for me you cannot contain
but somehow you always bring me pain
Oh what a tragedy!
that day you decided to deny my pregnancy
from me you decided to run
but I for you bore you your first son
See you indirectly, directly, threatened, suggested that
"If girl your love for me has no skin on skin sex
then you are at risk of being my ex"
So I did it, have done it, received it, now have it
Have HIV AIDS!

Tell me, what does it mean to love, what does it mean to love?
Today I tell you it comes from above
It's time we go back to the beginning bare basics love origin
I don't speak religion
just total submission
to the man upstairs

For in his word LOVE is clearly defined
and his love for you so big and bold can never be undermined

Fear the Lord is the beginning of all wisdom
Enter his kingdom
LOVE LOVE LOVE like Corinthians 13 says you must
In Jesus I will put my trust
I will not have sex
even if Baby I am at risk of being your ex
I will abstain
In God's love I will remain
there will be NO predictable predicted predictions of contradictions
contradicting this thing called LOVE.

Works Cited

Gräbner, Cornelia. "Performance Poetry: New Languages and New Literary Circuits?" *World Literature Today* 82.1 (January–February 2008, 21 paras, http://eprints.lancs.ac.uk/14200/1/Poetics_of_Performance_Poetry.pdf (accessed 13 January 2010).

Appendix 1

See samples of performance poetry from 'The Lover and Another' on YouTube:

Poet	URL
Nokwe Mchunu	http://www.youtube.com/watch?v=Js_NczP3eaA
Joy Dlamini	http://www.youtube.com/watch?v=GcW-6U269KM

Appendix 2
Handout

APPLIED ARTS FOR HIV/AIDS AWARENESS – AAA-HA!

RELATIONSHIPS AND MORE

RELATIONSHIPS AND MORE

The big deal at the moment is the issue of MULTIPLE CONCURRENT PARTNERSHIPS

This means having more than one partner at one time. No, not both at exactly the same time in the same place: but it's about having a lover and another lover undercover…..

The makhwapheni, the spare wheel, the small house, the second office … whatever you want to call it, it's the same thing.

This means that while a person may have a steady partner in a long-term relationship, they also have multiple partners on the outside. These partnerships usually overlap, forming a type of sexual network.

So what's wrong with that?

If one of the partners within a sexual network gets infected with HIV, the virus spreads rapidly to others, as HIV is most infectious during the first three to six weeks after infection.

According to a recent survey, 13% of young men and 4% of young women between the ages of 15–24, reported that they had concurrent partners. The survey also found that people in this age group have a greater chance of becoming involved with multiple and concurrent partners. In very plain terms, this means that it's very likely that this is happening on campus, and the more people you have sex with, the more chance there is of you being infected with HIV, and of you infecting others.

Multiple and concurrent partnerships may also involve the exchange of material goods and status between a man or a woman better off economically, and a younger partner who isn't. The younger partner is expected to give sexual favours in return to a sugar daddy or sugar mummy. Usually this means the younger or less powerful partner has no say in how sex is performed, whether it is with or without a condom, which means that they are more at risk of infection with HIV.

Multiple concurrent partnerships are the fastest way that HIV is spreading in South Africa.

What about condoms:

Well, in longer-term relationships, people seem to stop using condoms. This is usually linked to issues of trust and faithfulness …… but being in a long-term relationship does not always guarantee that there are just the 2 of you in the equation …..
SO THERE IS A LOT TO THINK ABOUT

RELATIONSHIPS TRUST FAITHFULNESS

All big words. But how do we understand them?

A relationship is a state of connectedness between people, and usually implies that there is an emotional connection. The emotional part is what makes relationship complicated!

Most relationship experts agree that a healthy relationship is based on the following:

Mutual respect

Respect in a relationship means that each person values who the other is and appreciates them! They also understand, and would never challenge, the other person's boundaries.

Trust

Trust means exposing your vulnerabilities to somebody, but believing that they will not take advantage of your openness. It's also about assessing the probabilities of gain and loss, and concluding that your partner will behave in a predictable manner.

Honesty

Honesty means not having to lie, and not being lied to, and not keeping secrets.

Support

In a healthy relationship, your partner should be there as a shoulder to cry on when you need it, and a person to celebrate with when you want to have fun!

Fairness

There needs to be a sense of equality in relationships; some give-and-take. Without this, a relationship can turn into a power struggle, with one person fighting to get his or her way all the time and the other person always giving in.

Separate identities

Relationships are made up of individuals who are different people. Keeping your sense of who you are beyond being "someone's partner" is important.

Communication

Talking, being open, and asking questions is the only way to make sure that the relationship stays on track. This also means spending some quality time together.

Faithfulness

Faithfulness is usually about the practice of living up to your commitments. If you make a promise and stick to it, then you are faithful to that promise. But what are you committing to?

Check out these websites for more info:
www.healthyplace.com
www.changingminds.com
www.thelife.com

Appendix 3
Rules

THE LOVER AND ANOTHER...

PERFORMANCE POETRY COMPETITION RULES

1. The competition is open to all registered students of UKZN, Pietermaritzburg.

2. Poems entered my be in any official South African language.

3. Poems must be original and performed by the writer.

4. Each contestant may enter no more than two poems.

4. Poets who enter two poems may win two prizes.

5. First, Second and Third prizes will be awarded. First Prize: R1 500, Second Prize R500, Third Prize R200

6. There is no entry fee for this contest.

7. Entry forms and the accompanying 'Relationships and More...' guidelines for the competition may be obtained at the Launch event, from the Drama Studies Office (Room 112 NAB) or downloaded from the UKZN /dramastudies website.

8. Contestants should submit a hard copy of the poem(s) with their entry form(s) to The Drama Studies Office, Room 112 New Arts Block.

9. Winners will be selected by a panel of judges at the Final Performance on August 20, 2009. The judges decision is final and no correspondence will be entered into.

10. Contestants will be judged on their performance and the originality, creativity and effectiveness of their communication of the ideas set out in the 'Relationships and More...' guidelines to this competition.

11. Prize money payment will be made once the winners have completed a payment form.

12. By entering the competition each poet agrees to release his or her name, likeness and poem for potential publicity purposes. All poems remain the property of the poet, but may be posted on the UKZN website, and used in a potential publication researching and or celebrating this event.

13. The organizers reserve the right to remove a poem from the competition for any reason.

⌘

SELLOANE MOKUKU

Do, Be, Do

Insights from 'Rapid Cognition' in a Theatre-Making Process

Introduction

THE WINTER/SUMMER INSTITUTE in Theatre for Development (WSI) is a biennial inter-university programme that brings together students and faculty members from diverse cultures and different countries for a residency under an established theme. The WSI has developed a method of playmaking that integrates and builds on a number of established methods in applied theatre. Furthermore, the focus is on deepening, enlarging, and refining the improvisational "tasks" offered by the staff/faculty. Subsequently, a play is devised where students/actors play multiple roles. As a pedagogical approach, its generative process uses techniques such as improvisation and spontaneity or 'theatre without script'[1] to create theatre that is experiential and experimental. This essay endeavours to unpack 'rapid cognition', a theory concerned with the ability to think instinctively, circumventing time and logic. Malcolm Gladwell maintains that the life experience that individuals possess has enough power to intuitively and rapidly guide them to correct understanding.[2] The making of WSI's 2008 play *It's Just You and Me, My Wife and Your Boyfriend/Ke 'Na le Uena, Mosali oa ka le Mohlan-*

[1] Jonathan Fox, *Acts of Service: Spontaneity, Commitment, Tradition in Nonscripted Theatre* (New York: Tusitala, 1994).

[2] Malcolm Gladwell, *Blink: The Power of Thinking Without Thinking* (Harmondsworth: Penguin, 2005).

kana oa Hau Feela, which embraced the residency theme of 'Power, Denial and HIV/ AIDS: Chances, Choices and Changes', will be used to illustrate seminal moments such as group work/tasks and reflections, where ideas were generated through 'rapid cognition'. Although 'rapid cognition' falls within the mode of the 'right hemisphere' of the brain, evidence in the WSI theatre-making approach suggests that it can be trained. The benefits of this would include heightened awareness in decision-making.

Defining 'Rapid Cognition'

The story goes that while taking a bath, the Greek mathematician Archimedes discovered the 'principle of buoyancy'.[3] He ran naked through the streets of Syracuse shouting "Eureka, Eureka!" As the story suggests, seeking an answer must have preoccupied Archimedes' mind and existence for some time before he suddenly knew the answer. This essay is concerned with facilitation of 'rapid cognition – the power of thinking without thinking', a theory that, Gladwell argues in *Blink*, is synonymous with the psychological term 'thin slicing', in the context of the WSI theatre-making process. Examples will be drawn from the WSI playmaking process mentioned.

'Rapid cognition' is concerned with the shortest form of knowing and thinking as opposed to long indecisive consideration because of a belief that one lacks enough information to make decisions. At the core of this theory are realizations that, at any given time, people, due to information and experience that accrue over time, have enough information to make informed decisions and choices – that a certain type of unconscious thinking is constant for human beings and may then result in moments of inspiration. This thinking is unpredictable; people just know it, without even knowing how, and they are often right. It appears to be based on experience and thoroughly internalized knowledge as well as on the safety of the context and the encouragement of spontaneity.

Given the unpredictability of responses or forms of behaviour that emanate from 'rapid cognition', there is resonance with social critical theory in rejecting the dualism that may be caused by distinguishing theory from practice. Thus the reasoning accustomed to science or positivist thinking is shifted to thinking that is more associated with instinct or interpretation, which also

[3] "Mathematics," http://maths.about.comm/library/blbioarchimedes.htm (accessed 5 September 2008).

challenges such notions as 'truth' and unsettles the power structures inherent in our acceptance of 'expertise'. Central to 'thin slicing' is "the ability of our unconscious to find patterns in situations and behaviour based on very narrow slices of experience."[4] The recognition of such patterns has a role in decision-making, especially in the WSI theatre-making process when groups have been assigned creative tasks that require swift resolution.

The *Daily Telegraph* journalist Sarah Sands maintains that 'rapid cognition' is "both liberating and dangerous":

> You know whether your hunch was right only in hindsight. Human creativity is a wonderful thing [...] and it is inextricably linked to human error.[5]

Gladwell is aware of this possible drawback. In this regard, two examples that may lead to the negative side of 'thin slicing' are observed. One is the phenomenon of the 'Warren Harding error', where judgments may be made on the basis of mere looks. The other one is the 'Implicit Association Test (IAT) tool' which suggests that people make more inherent connections "between pairs of ideas that are already related in our minds than we do between pairs of ideas that are unfamiliar to us."[6] It could be argued that these miscalculations are "at the root of a good deal of prejudice and discrimination,"[7] which is likely to betray our choices.

Betty Edwards argues that, of the two brain hemispheres (right and left), the right hemisphere is a mode concerned with "the intuitive, subjective, relational, holistic, time free mode," and has largely been ignored; the educational system has placed emphasis on the "verbal, rational, on the left hemisphere."[8] To this end, Gladwell argues that 'rapid cognition#, which would fall within the mode of the right hemisphere, can be taught and that "if we can control the environment in which rapid cognition takes place, then we can control rapid cognition."[9]

---

[4] Gladwell, *Blink*, 23.

[5] www.telegraph.co.za (accessed 12 November 2008).

[6] *Blink*, 77.

[7] *Blink*, 76.

[8] Betty Edwards, *Drawing on the Right Side of the Brain: How to Unlock Your Hidden Artistic Talent* (Los Angeles: J.P. Tarcher, 1979): 36.

[9] *Blink*, 253.

Methodology

To unpack the theory, qualitative research was used, particularly phenomenology, as a research method involving a choice of complementary methods such as focus-group discussion and diaries. This approach is concerned with the question of "what are the lived experiences of particular people."[10] In this instance, the focus is among and between the WSI participants (both faculty members and students). Mark Fortier notes the similarity to Judith Butler's use of phenomenology in a "feminist context by tracing the French feminist Simone de Beauvoir's assertion that one is not born, but becomes, a woman";[11] the WSI process provides an enabling environment for participants to embrace creativity and thus become catalysts. I believe that understanding their lived experience will guide in answering the facilitation of 'rapid cognition' in the WSI theatre-making. Myron Orleans explains that, in phenomenology,

> each actor assumes that every other actor knows what he or she knows of this world: All believe that they share common sense. However, each person's biography is unique, and each develops a relatively distinct stock of typifications and recipes. Therefore, interpretations may diverge.[12]

This explanation resonates well with social critical theory that recognizes the multiple truths which individuals perceive about issues. It is thus interesting to learn how meaning was negotiated in constructing a theatre piece with participants of varying age, economic, political, social, and cultural backgrounds.

WSI Philosophy

The Winter/Summer Institute (WSI) is both experiential and experimental and its facilitation approach views the representation of different cultures within the residency as a resource in the theatre-making process. Even though the medium of communication at the residency is English, there is freedom

---

[10] Brian Edmiston & Jeffrey Wilhelm, "Playing in Different Keys: Research Notes for Action Researchers and Reflective Drama Practioners," in *Researching Drama and Arts Education: Paradigms and Possibilities*, ed. Philip Taylor (London: Falmer, 1996): 90.

[11] Mark Fortier, *Theory/Theatre: An Introduction* (London: Routledge, 2nd ed. 2002): 45.

[12] http://hss.fullerton./edu/sociology/orleans/phenomenology.htm (accessed 7 February 2009).

during the creative process for participants to express themselves in any language or cultural expression. Students observed that

> It feels like when there wasn't that external uh… ok, run this scene, ok stop. Run this scene, no, no, no stop. Ok, wait. Change this… change this, and when that did not happen and we were just allowed to go through, and after we've gone through the fire and looked back and reflected on it then it felt like we owned it somehow and then we could go back and click, click, click, then we could see the shifts. (2008/WSI/FG[13])

As a pedagogical approach, the model relies on generating evocative material that creates a theatre piece by drawing on people's lived experiences and employing a variety of theatre techniques: semiotics, conventions, games, and improvisation. Also evident in the WSI theatre-making process is a focus on empowerment,[14] healing,[15] and 'rapid cognition', a theory concerned with the ability to think instinctively, circumventing time and logic . Thus individual experiences and knowledge become central to embracing the concept of 'transformative learning'.[16] In this regard, the environmentalist Michael Jackson posits that

> in explicit transformation learning exercises, activities can be planned that increase the intensity of cognitive dissonance by highlighting the contradictions and by exposing the manoeuvres by which the mind seeks an easy way out.[17]

The WSI Context

Since 2006, the WSI has been making theatre that elicits dialogue, thinking, and examination on topical issues. It thus provokes its residency participants and audience members to speak out and/or establish a platform for debate.

---

[13] FG refers to focus-group discussions.

[14] Augusto Boal, *Theatre of the Oppressed*, tr. Charles A. McBride, María-Odilia Leal McBride & Emily Fryer (*Teatro do oprimido e outras poéticas políticas*, 1975; tr. 1979; London: Pluto, 2002).

[15] Fox, *Acts of Service: Spontaneity, Commitment, Tradition in Nonscripted Theatre.*

[16] Carmel O'Sullivan, "Linking at the Equator Cross-Roads: 3rd World Congress of Drama, Theatre and Education," *Broadsheet* 15.1 (1999): 49–57.

[17] Michael Jackson, "Learning to think differently," *Southern African Journal of Environmental Education* 24 (2007): 85.

The WSI grew out of discussions between theatre practitioners, academics, and community-development initiators with a shared ownership of and commitment to community development. These discussions resulted in a collaborative proposal intended to enhance the capacity of students and staff in applied-theatre theory and practice, and to instigate an investigation of responsive and innovative ways to engage with HIV and AIDS through theatre.

The initiative brought together participants – students and teaching staff from the participating universities[18] – in a three-week residency on a chosen theme. The National University of Lesotho (NUL)'s Faculty of Humanities hosted the residency of the WSI.

The WSI residency structure consists of two weeks dedicated to the generation of work that culminates in a theatre piece, while the other week is spent working in collaboration with a chosen/given community. The participants are educators, facilitators, and actors, all of whom can potentially become trainers. According to the initiators, the WSI is developing a way to create collaborative group performance based on a phased structure of ensemble effort. The phases are as follows:

- Gathering information and accessing material;
- Generating improvisational responses to the material; and
- Shaping work for public performance (www.maketheatre.org).

The WSI integrates a number of already established methods and ideas charted by other theorists in applied drama and theatre. These are based predominantly on the pedagogy of Paulo Freire[19] and the praxis developed by Boal[20] in addition to local practices[21] based on the tradition in Africa of Theatre for Development. As indicated earlier, the WSI work is generated via

---

[18] Participating universities were the National University of Lesotho, University of Witwatersrand (Republic of South Africa) [School of Education], the University of Sunderland (UK) and the Empire State College, State University of New York (USA). The University of Sunderland was absent in 2008.

[19] Paulo Freire, *Pedagogy of the Oppressed*, tr. Myra Bergman Ramos (*Pedagogía del oprimido*, 1971; tr. 1972; Harmondsworth: Penguin, 1996).

[20] Augusto Boal, *Theatre of the Oppressed.*

[21] Examples are Marotholi Travelling Theatre (see Zakes Mda, *When People Play People: Development Communication Theatre* [Johannesburg: Wits UP & London: Zed, 1993]) and Liatla Productions, which uses mass media for therapy, education, and entertainment.

improvisation tasks, influenced by the work of Spolin and Johnstone.[22] The importance placed by these practitioners on spontaneity, on accepting 'offers' and not 'blocking', is congruent with the thinking of Gladwell. The practice of improvisation and the workings of rapid cognition have much in common, as students intimated:

> The facilitators would say…ok…can't talk…one, two, three…go into groups… you have 15 minutes to come up with something. (2008 /WSI/FG)

The tasks undertaken by participants during the SWI residency emanate from individual experiences, shared research, readings, presentations, and discussions, and this also created an opportunity for creativity.

> You knew everything, and that allowed a lot of space for creativity. You knew the important things, you knew how HIV worked or we did after the doctors had been with us, and that's sort of in your head. You don't have to constantly think about it, you incorporate it because it is there it's there, you know it, you incorporate it without having to try. (2008/WSI/FG)

The role of facilitation in enabling such processes is therefore crucial. In any given drama process the role of the facilitator(s) is dynamic, in that they are entrusted "to create an atmosphere of trust and synergy from which come results."[23] Given this situation, a need to trust the power of human knowledge accumulated through lived experience is pivotal. Through the skilful employment of different elements of drama, participants can be led towards a moment of insight or recognition when greater understanding is evoked. In a creative process, spontaneity and intuition are synonymous with 'rapid cognition'. For Spolin, improvisation enables the knowing of self and the environment differently; "through spontaneity we are re-formed into ourselves," and thus have an opportunity to "free [ourselves] from handed down frames of reference, memory choked with old facts and information and undigested theories and techniques of other people's findings."[24]

---

[22] Viola Spolin, *Improvisation for the Theatre: A Handbook of Teaching and Directing Techniques* (1963; Evanston IL: Northwestern UP, 3rd ed. 1999); Keith Johnstone, *Impro: Improvisation and the Theatre* (London: Eyre Methuen, 1981).

[23] Fran Rees, *The Facilitator Excellence Handbook: Helping People Work Creatively and Productively Together* (San Francisco: Jossey–Bass/Pfeiffer, 1998): 1.

[24] Spolin, *Improvisation for the Theatre*, 4.

The WSI process entails preparation by all participants. The first phase involves faculty only and the second phase involves all the participants as it pertains to the play-generation process. The figure below demonstrates this:

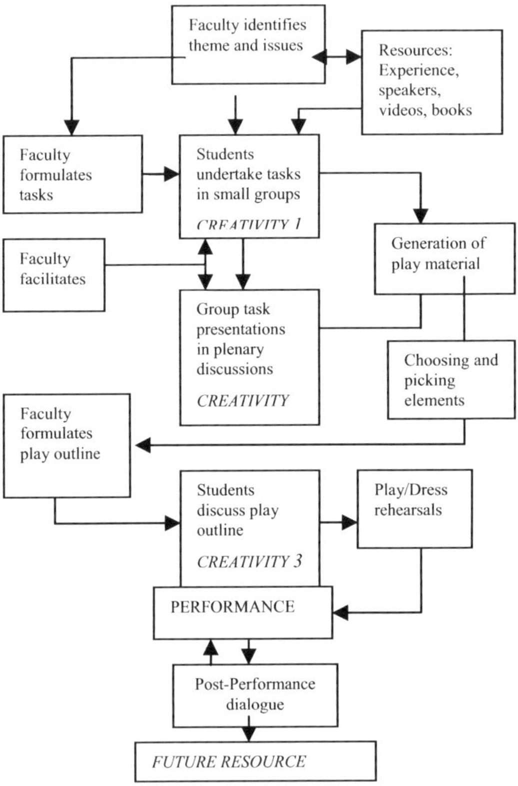

Figure 1: WSI Play-Generation Process

The Case of the WSI 2008 Play-Making Process

Preparation for the residency is a characteristic of the WSI. It takes place at two different levels. One precedes the residency, and the other occurs during it. Based on the plans of the faculty, students also engage in some preparations. Faculty members meet regularly during the residency to plan, think through, and rethink activities/creative tasks that can enhance the generation of material for the production of a play. Members normally share their experiences and, if these are found to be relevant, agree to use them as generative strategies.

Students prepare in order to equip themselves with adequate information to enable easier meeting with students and staff from other cultures. As indicated above, the chosen theme for 2008 was 'Power, Denial and HIV/AIDS: Chances, Choices and Changes'. Moreover, the preparations are carried out in order to create a pool of knowledge that grows collectively in the minds of the participants – so that, when the tasks (which are drawn directly from the presentations/screenings/readings) are devised, participants can draw on shared influences: everyone draws from the same common denominators, references, and ethos. Nevertheless, on the shared platform we've built, individual's lives and psyches and experiences also play a role.

Presentations by invited speakers are meant to provide up-to-date information on issues relevant to the chosen theme. Presenters cover matters relating to the theme of the residency. For example, one of the local medical doctors, Dr Khosi, made a presentation on the Lesotho government's response to HIV and AIDS, indicating the real-life challenges that people face, such as reluctance to use condoms even if people have full knowledge of the benefits thereof. A person living positively with AIDS also shared her experience.

The term 'tasks' was used to refer to activities carefully chosen to guide students in the process of devising a play. Faculty members meet and agree on the tasks to be given to students. Tasks are drawn directly from the presentations, films, readings and discussions (as highlighted above). They are of limited duration but, depending on the task/s, the time allotted can range from fifteen minutes to two hours. Tasks are normally given to a bigger group, and two faculty members are assigned or attached to each group. At the beginning, there is an attempt to keep members of the group rotating, and after about four tasks, the rotation is stopped and students begin to work in the same groups. The environment has thus emerged as important in enabling 'rapid cognition', as students from Wits confirmed:

> We were in a solace place far away from our homes, we were in groups, where we were made to feel safe, it was a safe place, the environment – em … I think it was like external variables came together to lay a platform to produce something quickly and something that was meaningful and something that could be adapted and changed, like quickly. (2008/WSI/FG)

Hence, the tasks that are given in the WSI enable participants to cross boundaries likely to be created. Participants are enabled to connect with one another on the human level, and to grow from such an interaction, without dwelling on the process. The discussions and reflections built into the process ensure that the group does not settle for mundane everyday activities. They are encouraged to engage intellectually, to question, they are also questioned, but not in a top-down manner, everything is negotiated. Facilitators are reported to have always probed instead of giving direction on how things have to be done. "What if…?" "How about…?" was the language facilitators used as opposed to "This should be done this way." or "No, you are wrong!"

In many ways, the creative process begins to be nurtured. Confidence – 'the secret to man's success'[25] – is built up. Participants begin to learn from one another, and faculty members begin to make note of presentations that might work theatrically if a play were to be devised. In a way, the presentation of tasks starts a bank of ideas to pick and choose from for the creative tasks and play-construction.

Reflection follows the presentation of tasks. During this time, everyone is encouraged to make comments on presentations. Later, group members are encouraged to share their working process and to respond to some of the issues raised by other participants. This phase of reflection normally involves robust engagement whereby participants' preconceived ideas may be challenged and new insights uncovered. One student, Pulane, confirms in her diary the importance of reflection to the creative process:

> I think there are a few reasons why we felt so free to act out the scene spontaneously. First of all, we were just "playing" with some ideas and there was no "right or wrong" answer. Secondly, we felt supported and accepted by the other students in our group. And thirdly, because we were given clear instructions and expectations from the faculty, we could set our intention. (2008/WSI/SUNY participant #2)

Throughout the residency, the WSI programme is interfaced with breaks for tea, lunch, and supper as well as for excursions. There are special nights that are also designated formally for socialization. These serve as breathers, since the residency can be very intense. Moreover, participants get an opportunity to extend informally the discussions on issues arising from the theatre-making process. Experience has shown that issues raised in such informal discussions sometimes end up being in the play. Moreover, Tankiso notes in his diary:

---

[25] Barack Obama, *Dreams from My Father* (Edinburgh: Canongate, 2008): 8.

> Healthy food as well as "day offs" gave a mind a free space for creativity. Simply because all work and no play makes it boring and blind each day. (2008/WSI/NUL participant # 3)

This becomes significant in a creative process such as the one offered by the WSI, as the theatre-piece is shaped by what participants bring to the space or process. The time for ideas to be processed by the unconscious seems to be important for making them available later as new and usable ideas – a form of rapid cognition. In theatre-making, this means that participants are free to explore all the various possibilities presented by the process. In other words, they are always in waiting.

Frances and Roland Bee believe that, in a learning environment,

> learners already have a great reservoir of knowledge and skills and that their job [as facilitators] is to surface that experience; they do a lot of listening to the delegates [participants].[26]

This observation correlates with Gladwell's point that the experiences of individuals have enough power to rapidly guide them to correct understanding. This correlation therefore leads me to ponder tenets of facilitation and 'rapid cognition' in theatre-making.

It has, I trust, emerged from thia essay that facilitators create an environment that ensures safety and freedom so that participants can explore and experiment. Respondents referred to this kind of experience as 'non judgmental', 'safe', where they knew that there were no 'wrong or right' answers. A space for the manifestation of multiple 'truths' was thus created, and appears to have brought confidence to participants, who, in turn, shared their lived experiences.

Lioli reports:

> Mè Sebolelo one day said to me Lioli, I am expecting to hear your praise poem, so by saying that she actually forced me to do something and then I made a poem. (2008/WSI/NUL participant # 4)

Lioli said this opportunity enhanced his confidence. Later, the praise poem was incorporated in the final play. This experience suggests that some structure or pressure is helpful in generating new ideas. Although this experience cannot be generic in theatre-making, it does open up debate on the usefulness of context in the creative process. If the play can be 'about us' as part of

---

[26] Frances & Roland Bee, *Facilitation Skills* (London: Chartered Institute of Personnel and Development, 1998): 4.

humanity, we are able to share similar and dissimilar experiences and feel our connectedness. This approach has made students more daring and free to try things out. Some students reported that they ended up doing things that they would not normally do, and this was credited to the spirit of sharing of ideas, thoughts and feelings that had been created at the WSI. When groups were given tasks to do, some participants expressed subtle 'competitiveness', but stemming from good intentions and faith that what was presented would improve the play.

Time limits had a positive effect on students; however short the time, knowing that they had to present something to other group members compelled them to come up with something worthwhile. It was during these intense moments that members had some excellent performances to share with the group. There was a realization that sometimes time was spent in arguments, but that when the moment for presentations came, devising a play was created on the spot and the results were often very powerful. Some members commented on the motivating importance of performing before an audience. The structure of giving a task, allowing students to work on their own, making presentations, and giving time for reflection is useful in validating shared group experiences.

This structure is also the result of the planning that the WSI faculty engages with before and during the residency. As facilitators they are attuned to the overall structure meant to elicit responsive material on the theme of the residency. Being sensitive to the fact that the residency itself has taken people out of their comfort zone is also important and can be seen as a catalyst which enhances the nurturing of a shared vision.

> Improvisation is intuition in action, a way to discover the muse and learn to respond to her call… we begin by that always surprising process of free invention in which we have nothing to gain and nothing to lose. The outpourings of intuition consist of a continuous, rapid flow of choice, choice, choice, choices.[27]

Building on the WSI 2008 theme, perhaps what is to be appreciated most is the fact that 'when we improvise with the whole heart, riding this flow, the choices and images open into each other so rapidly that we have no time to get scared and retreat from what intuition is telling us.'[28]

---

[27] Stephen Nachmanovitch, *Free Play: The Power of Improvisation in Life and the Arts* (New York: Tarcher Putnam, 1990): 41.

[28] Nachmanovitch, *Free Play*, 41.

During the preparations of the WSI, materials such as books, videos, and articles are selected and made accessible to the group. Presenters are also invited, and they, too, play a significant role in enriching the content of the discussions. Owing to the interdisciplinary nature of participants, they likewise regarded themselves as resources. For example, some people made use of their experience as counsellors to engage in content shaping the play. Some people reported that before coming to the residency, they engaged in a number of activities that would inform their participation at the WSI. Some registered for improvisation classes, learned Sesotho, and learned about Lesotho as well as HIV and AIDS.

It emerged that resources may also be prejudiced, and so an opportunity to criticize them added value to the material that went into the creative process. Apart from deriving the name of the play from one of the presentations, participants also reported on how they were inspired in the devising process by the information they gained from the presenters, books, or videos.

As argued earlier, the information and resources provided a body of knowledge and experience from which spontaneous decisions could be taken in the manner suggested by 'rapid cognition'.

Conclusion

It emerged that 'rapid cognition' requires thinking on one's feet. Although such spontaneity is clearly important in problem-solving and in responding flexibly to immediate input, this notion might be problematic if the group is not linguistically homogeneous.

From a theoretical perspective, the phenomenon of 'rapid cognition' is complex. Its manifestation requires individual knowledge, understanding, and experiences to engage responsively in any given context. However, the HIV and AIDS milieu throws up diverse dynamics to which the WSI is sensitive. Some of those include an appreciation of critical issues relating to health-belief models, the complexity of power in relation to gender in poverty, protocols in testing for and treating HIV and AIDS, as well as participants/facilitators' world-orientation. These are critical considerations, lest the proposed theory is viewed as anti-intellectual, idealistic, and simplistic – a situation that would be parochial in terms of what constitutes the knowledge-base and creativity in the WSI's theatre-making.

Knowledge that participants bring with them to the residency is rich enough to enable them to create credible work that will probably have a long-lasting impact on them. In my view, this is because, within a certain structure, participants are allowed to be experimental and explorative. Time pressure at the WSI does not allow for procrastination or for fear on the part of participants that they do not have enough knowledge. It confirms the idea that, at any given time, people have enough information to make informed decisions based on the interactions and experiences gained over their lifetime

Controlling the creative space lies at the core of enabling 'rapid cognition'. As shown in the study, the notion of controlling the environment opens up boundless opportunities for dialogue on topical issues. This correlates with Mda's undeniable assertion that

> The skills of acting can be learned though improvisation. Indeed the narrative itself can be structured though improvisations. People need to learn the skills in order to create theatre on their own in their continuous community through dialogue, but the path to this goal is not through scripted plays.[29]

In this regard, Gladwell notes:

> it doesn't seem like we have much control over whatever bubbles to the surface from our unconscious. But we do, and if we can control the environment in which rapid cognition takes place, then we can control rapid cognition.[30]

As argued earlier, the participants' experiences, information, and resources provided a body of knowledge and experience from which spontaneous decisions could be taken in the manner suggested by 'rapid cognition'. The participants were encouraged to be explorative and just 'do' and to 'be' themselves within a theatre-making process. I believe that this recognition is in keeping with what Boal calls the "rehearsal for revolution."[31]

WORKS CITED

Bee, Frances, & Roland Bee. *Facilitation Skills* (London: Chartered Institute of Personnel and Development, 1998).

Boal, Augusto. *Theatre of the Oppressed*, tr. Charles A. McBride, María–Odilia Leal McBride & Emily Fryer (*Teatro do oprimido e outras poéticas políticas*, 1975; tr. 1979; London: Pluto, 2002).

---

[29] Mda, *When People Play People*, 23.

[30] *Blink*, 252–53.

[31] Boal, *Theatre of the Oppressed*, 141.

Edmiston, Brian, & Jeffrey Wilhelm. "Playing in Different Keys: Research Notes for Action Researchers and Reflective Drama Practioners," in *Researching Drama and Arts Education: Paradigms and Possibilities*, ed. Philip Taylor (London: Falmer, 1996): 85–96.

Edwards, Betty. *Drawing on the Right Side of the Brain: How to Unlock Your Hidden Artistic Talent* (Los Angeles: J.P. Tarcher, 1979).

Fox, Jonathan. *Acts of Service: Spontaneity, Commitment, Tradition in Nonscripted Theatre* (New York: Tusitala, 1994).

Fortier, Mark. *Theory/Theatre: An Introduction* (London: Routledge, 2nd ed. 2002).

Freire, Paulo. *Pedagogy of the Oppressed*, tr. Myra Bergman Ramos (*Pedagogía del oprimido*, 1971; tr. 1972; Harmondsworth: Penguin, 1996).

Gladwell, Malcolm. *Blink: The Power of Thinking Without Thinking* (Harmondsworth: Penguin, 2005).

Jackson, Michael. "Learning to think differently," *Southern African Journal of Environmental Education* 24 (2007): 82–89.

Johnstone, Keith. *Impro: Improvisation and the Theatre* (London: Eyre Methuen, 1981).

"Mathematics," http://maths.about.com/library/blbioarchimedes.htm (accessed 5 September 2008).

Mda, Zakes. *When People Play People: Development Communication Through Theatre* (Johannesburg: Wits UP & London: Zed, 1993).

Nachmanovitch, Stephen. *Free Play: The Power of Improvisation in Life an the Arts* (New York: Tarcher Putnam, 1990).

Obama, Barack. *Dreams from My Father* (Edinburgh: Canongate, 2008).

Orleans, Myron. "Phenomenology," in *Encyclopedia of Sociology*, http://hss.fullerton.edu/sociology/orleans/phenomenology.htm (accessed 7 February 2009).

O'Sullivan, Carmel. "Linking at the Equator Cross-Roads: 3rd World Congress of Drama, Theatre and Education," *Broadsheet* 15.1 (1999): 49–57.

Rees, Fran. *The Facilitator Excellence Handbook: Helping People Work Creatively and Productively Together* (San Francisco: Jossey–Bass/Pfeiffer, 1998).

Spolin, Viola. *Improvisation for the Theatre: A Handbook of Teaching and Directing Techniques* (1963; Evanston IL: Northwestern UP, 3rd ed. 1999).

⌘

JOHANNES VISSER

Space and Involvement

Theatre in (a) South African Prison

Introduction

THIS ESSAY WILL TAKE THE FORM of a 'Report to the Academy'[1] on work in progress. It should not be seen as a definitive research project but, rather, a sharing of ideas and observations. We can not yet provide answers or outcomes to all the questions that we stumbled upon during the research, but can begin to examine the process and investigate preliminary findings and experiences.

Although one of the focal points of this volume, it is impossible for me to isolate the HIV/AIDS issue. During our engagement with the Pretoria C-Max prison, we discovered that it is necessary to unravel a spider's web of surrounding issues, covering (among others) violence, rape, sexual activities, gang activities, and drug abuse – all related to, and inter-connected with, the problem of HIV and AIDS.

The basics of 'Theatre in Prison' may stay constant – but it is possible, through engaging with other disciplines (in this case the University of Pretoria's Departments of Social Work, Criminology, and Psychology, as well as the Centre for the Study of AIDS – CSA) to explore new ways of packaging the application of the theory and methods of applied theatre.

[1] Franz Kafka, *Report to the Academy* (1917), rev. ed. tr. Ian Johnston (Nanaimo, British Columbia: Malaspina University College, 2007).

A small space or fissure exists between the practised smile and the panoptic eye of the criminal,[2] where applied theatre may be able to forge a little bit of freedom in order to challenge authority. Hence the title of this essay.

The context in which this essay is situated refers to the notion of change within specific cultures. The high arts as well as popular culture underlie and feed into human and societal values and to the expression of these values. But what happens in a culture when the oppressed develops into the oppressor and, in turn, becomes the oppressed again? During her keynote address, Prof Claire Penn quoted Augusto Boal in stating that we can be both oppressor and oppressed at the same time.[3] I would like to pose a counter-position: the individual and/or community is constantly in flux between oppressors and oppressed. We all take on the role of either, as and when it suits us.

Focusing on the idea of theatre for/with/by the oppressed, it is of the utmost importance that drama and theatre in prison find new ways to transcend new kinds of repression, oppression, exploitation, and injustice.

Our research investigates the idea of applied theatre's ability to create a space of freedom within a system of formalized power, trying also to explore the space between 'us' and 'them'.

With reference to the interdisciplinary research and work done by the Drama Department in collaboration with the Department of Social Work and Criminology, the Department of Psychology, and the CSA, I must agree with what Hazel Barnes commented on in her response to Claire Penn's keynote address in the context of the conference on which the present volume is based: this type of collaboration provides fresh stimulus to action for all agents involved, not only the students and staff members of the different departments but also the wardens and inmates of the male juvenile pre-trial section of the C-Max prison in Pretoria.

⌘

---

[2] Cf. Baz Kershaw, "Pathologies of Hope in Drama and Theatre," in *Theatre in Prison: Theory and Practice*, ed. Michael Balfour (Bristol & Portland OR: Intellect, 2004): 35.

[3] Claire Penn, "Drama, Doctors and HIV/AIDS," keynote address (Drama For Life, Africa Research Conference, Wits University, 2009).

Context

In the type of work we do, I personally feel that it is impossible to work for change and development without taking aspects of culture into consideration. Cultural identity can be developed by various groups (communities) both minority and majority.

> Traditionally culture could be seen as a factor of resistance, an opponent to change. The 'traditional ways' of the past could be perceived, especially by younger generations, as an obstacle to overcome in the process of achieving socio-political change. [...] The reason for this lies in the fact that culture provides any given community with a way to deal with sudden (and at times unwanted) changes. Current attempts to define culture start from a critical deconstruction of the past.[4]

The past has to make sense in an ever-changing present, and fortunately culture is certainly changeable/adaptable. Therefore, applied theatre, as a tool for change, has a place in a community such as the prison environment. We need to engage with this community with its strong sense of identity to be able to bring about any change in behaviour, for this is a cultural issue.

A common complaint among mostly white South Africans is that there is too much emphasis on blaming the legacy of apartheid for the problems of the present. "Why can't we put all that behind us, forgive and forget and move on?"[5] Blaming the past will not solve the problems of the present.

This does not mean that the rapist or the murderer can avoid all moral responsibility by blaming apartheid. The problem is that many such offenders have no sense of moral responsibility in the first place. And *that* is the legacy of apartheid – the *culture* of rape and other acts of violence, gangsterism, substance abuse, and numerous other sub-cultures.

The policy of apartheid deliberately set out to destroy family life in the name of an ideology. Generations of children grew up fatherless and often motherless as well. And children deprived of parental love in infancy find it much more difficult to form loving relationships with other people as they grow up. Apartheid created several generations of children like this, and now AIDS is creating several more, as the number of child-headed households is

---

[4] Kees Epskamp, *Theatre for Development: An Introduction to Context, Applications & Training* (London & New York: Zed, 2006): 29–30.

[5] Anon., "The legacy of apartheid and the culture of violence," *Khanya* (4 November 2007), http://khanya.wordpress.com/2007/11/04/the-legacy-of-apartheid-and-the-culture-of-violence/ (accessed 24 October 2009).

growing all the time. South Africa is so overwhelmed by violence that it has indeed become a way of life, a *culture* which has dangerous consequences, especially for our youth.

Apartheid left a legacy of poverty, inequality, and a sense of the nobility of violence in the struggle to end an oppressive system.[6] The political transition ushered in uncertainty and more crime. There was already a willingness, deeply embedded in South African society, to use violence to solve fairly minor disputes.

South Africa's youth (specifically black youth) also had high expectations that democracy would bring more jobs and a better quality of life. That hasn't happened. In some cases they have taken out their disillusionment and anger by turning to crime.

Looking at violence, rape, and HIV/AIDS, it is impossible to separate them from gender relations, particularly in the South African context, and the expression of violence against women has to be viewed in this specific political context. One of the most striking features of South African society is its stratification along class, race, and gender lines. One may be able to accept that violence and abuse against women is a manifestation of the imbalance of power inherent in patriarchal relations. In the South African socio-political context, where the working-class see themselves as oppressed and impotent, their frustration at this marginalization is likely to take expression in violence and oppression in the private domain, where women are mostly the target.[7]

While the term 'culture of violence' indicates the broad acceptability of aggression, there are differences in the extent to which certain groups endorse it. Gangs are an example of a subculture in which violence is particularly pronounced, and this is connected to the composition of its members and their location within society. First, with regard to township gangs, both the youth and the 'maleness' of their members encourage the use of violence, as a result of its strong association with masculinity. Secondly, given the marginalization of the members, violence offers a quick and easy method to level the social playing-field, to make an impression on an otherwise indifferent society, to gain social approval (from fellow members), and to obtain power and pleasure. Given the deterioration of moral codes in South Africa, men are also more likely to rape, as there are fewer social and legal restraints. They are

---

[6] "The legacy of apartheid and the culture of violence."

[7] Carolyn Dempster, "Guns, gangs and culture of violence," *BBC News* (10 April 2002), http://news.bbc.co.uk/2/hi/africa/1919382.stm (accessed 25 October 2009).

able to engage in gang or individual rape, with the confidence that their crime is unlikely to be reported and that, even if it were, they are unlikely to be arrested and convicted.[8]

We must keep in mind that the criminal identity is created by the biological basis, individual development, and social context, each in relationship with the others and none of them fixed – the criminal may be viewed by some as being at the extreme end of society. But then, James Thompson states that the study of law-breakers is at the same time a study of the law-makers. A study of the prison is a study of the society in which it exists. He quotes Winston Churchill as saying (already in 1911):

> the mood and temper of the public in regard to the treatment of crime and criminals is one of the most unfailing tests of the civilisation of any country [...] the treatment of crime and criminals make and measure the stored up strength of a nation and are sign and proof of the living virtue in it.[9]

In doing what we do, we must strive to connect with those forgotten/invisible voices (black and white) who, despite their crimes, come with the same cultural, political, and social bonds as ourselves – both during and after apartheid.

Question

The question we constantly ask ourselves in this endeavour is: How can we get involved, how can we best utilize the cultural practices of applied drama and theatre to fill the void, or to create a positive space for change and development within institutions with formalized power?

Methodology

When working with theatre in prison, it is not always imperative to create an academic construct for the work to fit into; it is sometimes more important to listen to the story, to hear the telling of an experience.

---

[8] Carolyn Dempster, "Guns, gangs and culture of violence"; Anon., "Highest incidence of rape – a 'culture of violence' (South Africa)," *WIN News* (22 March 1998), http://www.highbeam.com/doc/1G1-20756740.html (accessed 25 October 2009).

[9] James Thompson, *Applied Theatre: Bewilderment and Beyond* (Bern: European Academic, 2003): 9–10.

I want to quote Balfour again for emphasis:

> between the practised smile and the panoptic eye, between the politician and the policeman, between human rights and legalised oppression, in any system designed by some to control others there will always be a space for resistance, a fissure in which to forge at least a little freedom.[10]

Grasping this creative space cannot be of use without grappling with the oppressive systems – the prison, the ideology which seeks to eliminate 'them'. That is why creative work is customarily an unwelcome challenge to authority.

Research methods included the following:

— Participatory action research in creation and documentation of personal stories and experiences done by the Department of Criminology;
— trend and change analysis in follow-up sessions by Psychology's postgraduate students;
— consultation of existing literature – to equip students with knowledge and insight regarding the nature, causes, and incidence of juvenile delinquency – learning that the various circumstances of the individual must be taken into account – thus, not to be judgmental in interviews, conversations, and the creation of performances;
— making use of the knowledge of experts: Karen Booyens from the Department of Psychology, a well-known academic in the field of criminology, Reineth Prinsloo of the Department of Social Work and Criminology; and Johan Maritz of the CSA, among others;
— excursions to Pretoria Local Remand Detention Centre provided the opportunity to get acquainted with spatial settings in which performances took place, as well as introducing the students to the unique dialect/slang of the juvenile detainees, to enable them to use this in the creation of performances; and
— making use of the completed questionnaires and preparatory reports one compiled by the Departments of Criminology and Psychology to assess the needs of the community.

[10] Balfour, "Introduction" to *Theatre in Prison: Theory and Practice*, ed. Balfour, 5.

The Performances

From 2006 to 2009 staff and students of the Drama Department were involved in the development of at least sixteen performances dealing with the issue of HIV/AIDS, with at least half of these performances delivered to juvenile trial-awaiting detainees in the Pretoria C-Max institution.

Before discussing a few aspects of the performances devised by the Drama Department, it could be enlightening to share some statistics about the audience and partners we had to cater for. As indicated above, this information was gained from our research in collaboration with the Departments of Psychology, Social Work, and Criminology as well as the Centre for the Study of AIDS.[11]

By July 2007, the C-Max prison in Pretoria (including the Remand Detention Centre) was overcrowded by 220%. Fortunately this had dropped to 175% by June 2009 – but, of course, this remains a nagging problem.

As far as the age of juvenile detainees is concerned, 45 % are between the ages of 15 and 19, with 55% over the age of 20. 74% have obtained an educational level between grades 7 and 11, with only 18% achieving grade 12.

Looking at religious concerns, 57% were Christians, with Islam at 15%, 8% non-religious, and 20% adhering to other religions. Enquiries into the duration of the detention period before trial disclosed that at least 26% of the group had been detained for a year or longer.

During the needs assessment of the group we found that the most pressing physical needs included beds, sheets, and blankets as well as hygienic commodities like shampoo, washing powder, toothbrushes, and toothpaste, and, most importantly – toilet paper. 50% of the detainees had only one set of clothes; 25% claimed that they had no free access to medical attention; 48% had no contact with the outside world (lack of phone cards or phone booths); and 44% do not get any financial aid from relatives or guardians.

As far as socio-emotional needs are concerned, 46% do not receive visits at all. When asked whether the individual had someone to trust and talk to in the prison environment, 62% replied that they could confide in friends, relatives, social workers and wardens; 38% did not feel they had this opportunity.

---

[11] S. Van den Berg, "Intervention with Communities: Report on Needs Assessment Done in Pretoria Local Remand Detention Centre with Children and Juveniles Awaiting Trial" (unpublished document for MWP 261: Social Work in Practice; Reineth Prinsloo, Department of social Work and Criminology, University of Pretoria, 2008).

Almost 70% of the detainees indicated that they would like to take part in group sessions and workshops to be able to freely discuss their fate and lives. Participation in these groups to receive information about specific life-skills amounted to the following:

Anger management – 85%
HIV/AIDS – 83%
Self-esteem – 76%
Conflict handling – 73%

44% of the detainees expressed concerns about their own safety in the prison environment; and, as far as their feeling and attitudes about being detained goes, 84% expressed a feeling of regret, 57% felt remorse, 52% were sad about their circumstances, and only 2,7% wished to apologize for their actions.

From the detainees who expressed concerns about their perception of a lack of security and general well-being, the reasons for their statements were recorded as follows:

- Insufficient sleep (sleep deprivation)
- Beaten when sleeping
- Miss relatives
- Bad smell
- Physical and verbal abuse
- Don't like the place
- Fear
- It is not home
- Interpersonal conflict
- People are rough and violent
- Violence and murder
- Overcrowding and intimidation

Working in and with this community, and being surrounded by these circumstances, often left our students drained of emotion. Working with the Psychology Department, we could, fortunately, send them (or those who needed it) for debriefing and counselling after each contact session and/or performance. Also taxing on the emotional and energy resources of the students was the fact that as both groups gained more confidence and relaxed into newly established group dynamics, some of the inmates did get attached to the 'researchers' or 'performers'.[12] The student (or students) entering the facility and interacting with the community may be the first 'power' figure or 'outsider' taking interest in them personally and not in what they have done.

In the Drama Department we are in the fortunate position that the demographics of our student body is such that it enabled us to understand and deal with almost all of the different languages or dialects of the specific community. This communication enabled the community to share their stories and histories with the students of all the departments involved.

After the initial research, the drama students then start exploring scenarios, structures, actions, and options to develop stories aesthetically into performances.

In our specific project, the third-year students conceptualize the performances, and they are then allocated a group of second-year acting students (and in quite a few cases from community performance groups) to workshop their concepts and visions. Over a four-to-five-week period, they explore possibilities of engaging with the prison community. They create, refine, deconstruct, and re-refine the performance in close collaboration with us as staff members and also with their 'clients' or working partners – being Psychology, Social Work, Criminology, and the CSA. Daily progress reports are expected from them, as well as weekly viewings and at least three drafts of the developed script.

Working with a young audience implies high-energy performances, including (apart from acting) dance, physical theatre, and, of course, music and song, which normally provides the opportunity for interactive participation by both performers and inmates. (In 2008 we actually had a performance with the title *AIDS the Musical*, which was also performed on the UP campus, at the Department of Housing's HIV/AIDS conference, schools in the Tshwane metro, and at the Drama for Life Festival.)

On request by Psychology and Social Work, 2009's performances also made use of much more 'humour' than those of the previous three years. We experienced (as Jamie McLaren Lachman also pointed out during his 'Clowns Without Borders' workshop[13]) that a special bond can be forged between the

---

[12] Cf. Thompson, *Applied Theatre: Bewilderment and Beyond*, 172–73.

[13] Jamie McLaren Lachman, "Clowns Without Borders: Using Storytelling, Drama and Play Therapy for Psychosocial Interventions in Communities Affected by HIV AIDS in Southern Africa – Pathways to Empathetic Locally Sustainable Care"

separate individuals and groups when applying humour to an otherwise serious, and even grave, interaction. This also helps to share sensitive issues in ways that do not cause offence.

Of course, we did experience extreme reactions such as raucous laughter, clapping, stamping on chairs and the floor, wolf whistles, and even comments shouted at the performers. This usually happens as soon as a female performer enters the acting space, during scenes of either intimacy or physical violence, and, most of all, in scenes and actions depicting any form of sexual activity. After consulting with some of the audience members, the authorities, and researchers from the Department of Psychology, we found that these types of reaction normally stem from the recognition of the character, the scenario, or the action.

Certain structures can be created in anticipation of these extreme reactions. For example, in one of the performances in 2009 a brutal rape-scene was constructed and choreographed, with the perpetrator isolated on one side of the performance space and the victim on the other side (with precise coordination of movement, action, and reaction). During a question-and-answer session after the performance, it became clear that the act, the image, the 'message' was conveyed to the audience as effectively as it would have should the two characters have had physical contact. I would (personally) like to express admiration for the drama students for being daring, for being brutally honest in dealing with acts of rape, gang-rape, substance abuse, violence, and sodomy, in one case even depicting the delivery of drugs by storing it in the anal cavity.

Allow me a few remarks on the process of character-creation. As mentioned before, characters are devised directly from the stories and histories of individual members of the community. A few specific examples include:

- A substance abuser who turned to this practice as result of being raped by an uncle
- A gang member who killed the man who abused his mother
- A 'fictional' character who committed suicide after being gang raped.

In 2009, for the first time, we encountered the use of abstraction in the communication of individual, personal experiences or narratives. Thus, in one of

---

(workshop presented at the Drama for Life Africa Research Conference in Applied Drama & Theatre, Wits University, 2009).

the performances the characters illustrated different aspects of the same person (both offender and victim):

— The 'good' conscience
— The 'bad' conscience
— The heart
— The lungs
— The sexual organs
— The substance.

A significant learning experience was achieved by both parties involved, the inmates as well as the drama students. As illustration, I would like to conclude with a few remarks from our students:[14]

— "The work opened up new viewpoints – it is challenging but also liberating"
— "It taught me tolerance with, and acceptance of people differing from my self"
— "What we experienced smashed our own egos"
— "We taught by learning. We had to scrutinize our own ideologies as the audience became our equals."

Conclusion

What matters in the impact of the performance is not necessarily its overall message or 'lesson', but the opportunity given for the expression of a multiplicity of voices which normally would have been suppressed by the institution. But taking into account the complexities we deal with – we still have to ask: what have we really done? What opportunities have we unearthed to construct an alternative to existing ideologies? Were we able to create a space in which the construction of lives can be experienced?[15]

Factors/aspects/activities to take into account for increased success of this engagement with the specific community include:

— further intersectional and inter disciplinary cooperation to combine subjects such as health care in general, HIV/AIDS, anger-manage-

---

[14] Unpublished journals compiled for assessment by third-year students (Department of Drama, University of Pretoria, 2009).

[15] Kershaw, "Pathologies of Hope in Drama and Theatre," 39–40.

ment, self-worth, identity, sexuality, drug use and abuse, and a multitude of other problems and needs experienced;
— follow-up: success through short-term results offers no guarantee in the long run that participants will benefit from this type of project or programme – we must interactively engage with Sociology, Criminology, and the CSA doing the follow-up workshops and activities;
— long-term thinking: instead of yearly short-term, isolated projects – we have to look at long-term continuous engagement that is future-oriented;
— obtaining permission from the Department of Correctional Services to allow us to document (audio and audiovisual) contact between the parties involved in the specific institution.

Currently, our involvement is still a project *for* the community. We still have to explore the possibilities of creating continuous programmes *with* the community, and eventually *by* the community.

As a final comment I would like to agree with Kershaw's statement that they (our audience as well as the students) may not yet have achieved freedom – and have not yet had the opportunity) to actively and critically engage with the formal systems of power;[16] but we may have opened up the space to realize that such engagements may be possible.

WORKS CITED

Anon. "Highest incidence of rape – a 'culture of violence' (South Africa)," *WIN News* (22 March 1998), http://www.highbeam.com/doc/1G1-20756740.html (accessed 25 October 2009).

Anon. "The legacy of apartheid and the culture of violence," *Khanya* (4 November 2007), http://khanya.wordpress.com/2007/11/04/the-legacy-of-apartheid-and-the-culture-of-violence/ (accessed 24 October 2009).

Balfour, Michael. "Introduction" to *Theatre in Prison: Theory and Practice*, ed. Balfour (Bristol & Portland OR: Intellect, 2004): 1–18.

Dempster, Carolyn. "Guns, gangs and culture of violence," *BBC News* (10 April 2002), http://news.bbc.co.uk/2/hi/africa/1919382.stm (accessed 25 October 2009).

Epskamp, Kees. *Theatre for Development: An Introduction to Context, Applications & Training* (London & New York: Zed, 2006).

---

[16] Kershaw, "Pathologies of Hope in Drama and Theatre," 49.

Kafka, Franz. *Report to the Academy* (1917), tr. Ian Johnston (Nanaimo, British Columbia: Malaspina University College, 2007).

Kershaw, Baz. "Pathologies of Hope in Drama and Theatre," in *Theatre in Prison: Theory and Practice*, ed. Michael Balfour (Bristol & Portland OR: Intellect, 2004): 35–52.

Lachman, Jamie McLaren. "Clowns Without Borders: Using Storytelling, Drama and Play Therapy for Psychosocial Interventions in Communities Affected by HIV AIDS in Southern Africa – Pathways to Empathetic Locally Sustainable Care" (workshop presented at the Drama for Life Africa Research Conference in Applied Drama & Theatre, Wits University, 2009).

Penn, Claire. "Drama, Doctors and HIV/AIDS," keynote address (Drama For Life, Africa Research Conference, Wits University, 2009).

Thompson, James. *Applied Theatre: Bewilderment and Beyond* (Bern: European Academic, 2003).

——, ed. *Prison Theatre: Perspectives and Practice* (London & New York: Jessica Kingsley, 1998).

Unpublished journals compiled for assessment by third-year students (Department of Drama, University of Pretoria, 2009).

Van den Berg, S. "Intervention with Communities: Report on Needs Assessment Done in Pretoria Local Remand Detention Centre with Children and Juveniles Awaiting Trial" (unpublished document for MWP 261: Social Work in Practice; Reineth Prinsloo, Department of Social Work and Criminology, University of Pretoria, 2008).

⌘

Innovations in Research Practice/Theory

ALEXANDRA SUTHERLAND

Dramatic Spaces in Patriarchal Contexts

Constructions and Disruptions of Gender in Theatre Interventions About HIV

CAN THEATRE MAKE A DIFFERENCE, and if so, how? The research on which this essay was partly based intended to show how discrete moments of engaging young people through theatre can catalyse them into questioning gendered assumptions which drive mythologies, stigmas, and prejudices relating to HIV. This is based on my belief as a practitioner that applied-theatre approaches can create potentially transgressive spaces, a series of artistic transformations, where questions about entrenched stories and identities can be asked – particularly about what it might mean to be a man or a woman in an age of HIV. Jonothan Neelands has framed the overriding, nagging question I have: "What is more difficult to know is whether these artistic transformations can be said to also affect the broader socio-cultural domain."[1]

Implicit in much applied-theatre praxis is the hope that it can, particularly as many of these practices draw from or resonate with the theoretical terrain of cultural studies and, by extension, critical or liberatory pedagogy. Recent critiques of critical theory and pedagogy argue that, as an approach, its reduction to binaries of oppressor and oppressed is limiting and has not actually resulted in the liberation of the groups/communities it intends to. Elizabeth

[1] Jonothan Neelands, "Miracles are happening: beyond the rhetoric of transformation in the Western traditions of drama education," *RiDE: Research in Drama Education* 9.1 (2004): 50.

Ellsworth argues that key terms associated with critical pedagogy and, also to be noted, applied-theatre practices, "such as 'empowerment', 'student voice', 'dialogue', and even the term 'critical' – are repressive myths that perpetuate relations of domination."[2] In the South African context, Jonathan Jansen draws on Ellsworth's argument,[3] maintaining that critical theory and pedagogy are fundamentally limiting in a post-conflict society like South Africa:

> Critical theory both conceives and constructs the world as divided between black and white, the working classes and the privileged classes, legal citizen and illegal immigrant, men and women, straight and queer, oppressors and oppressed; its dialogical pretences notwithstanding, the world is taken as torn among rival groups.[4]

The critique of critical theory is that it glosses over the complexities of power, and cannot accommodate "the multiple, contradictory, overlapping social positions not reducible either to race, or class, or gender."[5] Classrooms are sites of rival spaces, contending histories, and lived experiences. Jansen argues for a post-conflict pedagogy which recognizes and can account for the pain and trauma of both sides, through the creation of sustained discursive spaces which can provide a safe site for the playing-out of a multiplicity of identities. It seems that drama and theatre are uniquely positioned to create and support the context-specificity of each group and the particular narratives and identities that each group brings to the space. Within a gender-based drama programme, it is unhelpful to construct men as bad and women as victims, despite the statistical reality that young women really are the biggest victims of the AIDS pandemic. However, the young people I worked with automatically constructed men as bad and women as victims when first asked to create images of 'man' and 'woman'. Not only does this give a very clear picture of what is going on in this context for this group of young people in relation to how roles of men and women are conceived, but it also allows for drama processes which can interrupt what Jansen calls "received knowledge."

---

[2] Elizabeth Ellsworth, "Why Doesn't This Feel Empowering? Working Through the Repressive Myths of Critical Pedagogy," *Harvard Educational Review* 59.3 (August 1989): 298.

[3] According to Ellsworth, many terms associated with critical pedagogy become ahistorical and depoliticized abstractions.

[4] Jonathan D. Jansen, "On the Clash of Martyrological Memories," *Perspectives in Education* 27.2 (June 2009): 150.

[5] Ellsworth, "Why Doesn't This Feel Empowering?," 302.

Jansen argues for a pedagogy of hope, where counter-narratives are shown so as not to essentialize social positions of oppressor and oppressed. In these workshops, the simple act of asking 'if you could change something about this image, what would you change?' enacts a different possibility – and does not insist on changing only the position of the oppressed, as it recognizes that power shifts, as does oppression. In these cases, boys often changed the role of men by putting babies in their arms. This embodied, live gesture performs the multiplicity of possibilities of what it might mean to be a man.

Why Focus on Gender?

> Because… its there. And it impacts on every interaction whether we are conscious of it or not. It's not the only thing that impacts on human interactions but it is a significant factor and often an invisible or unnoticed one.[6]

The reasons for the huge gender inequalities that exist in South Africa are multi-faceted, and relate to complex historical, cultural, and social processes. It is these gender inequalities that are now recognized as one of the primary drivers of social diseases such as HIV/AIDS.

On the one hand, women are appropriated in the 'new' South Africa as symbols of national strength and endurance in mainstream nation-building efforts and women's rights and equality are guaranteed by the constitution.[7] However, the role and treatment of women outside of this imagined nation is radically different. Gross inequalities exist, particularly within intimate settings, which are often dominated by gender-based violence. In this context it is naive and ignorant to preach condom use and abstinence as means of combatting HIV, when women often have very little negotiating power in sexual relations.

Statistically, gender and poverty determine the likelihood of contracting HIV. Young women (ages 15 to 29) have the *highest risk* of new HIV infections in South Africa: women and girls between the ages of 15 and 24 ac-

---

[6] Sharon Grady, "Feminist methodology," in *Research Methodologies for Drama Education*, ed. Judith Ackroyd (Stoke-on-Trent: Trentham, 2006): 82.

[7] Ulrike Kistner, *Gender-Based Violence and HIV/AIDS in South Africa: A Literature Review* (Johannesburg: CADRE, 2003).

counted for 32% of all new infections.[8] Young women in this age group are six times more likely to catch HIV than young men in the same age group. This group also has the highest risk of rape, yet the links between gender-based violence and HIV issues have only been theorized and documented fairly recently.[9] Women are physically, socially, and culturally far more vulnerable to HIV infection than men.

Gender determines

- how/whether one chooses an intimate partner;
- deciding whether to disclose status;
- deciding whether to go for VCT;
- how to communicate results to others;
- how one reacts if one's intimate partner discloses their HIV test;
- how/whether one can negotiate safe sex & condom usage; and
- deciding who cares for person with HIV.[10]

Yet it is men who are driving the spread of HIV through patriarchal and often deeply misogynistic practices embedded in a concept of masculinity which is intricately connected with the number of sexual conquests one has, and the unquestioned authority and control over women, who are seen as property to be bought, owned, controlled, and defended.[11]

AIDS is a social epidemic, and any disease is given meaning through social processes:

> It acquires meaning and significance from its human context, from the ways in which it infiltrates the lives of the people, from the reactions it provokes, and from the manner in which it gives expression to cultural and political values.[12]

Applied theatre, as a socially based artform which aims to construct meaning through performance processes, can therefore shape and contest some of the

---

8 Human Sciences Research Council (2005).

9 Kistner, *Gender-Based Violence and HIV/AIDS in South Africa: A Literature Review.*

10 *Gender-Based Violence and HIV/AIDS in South Africa: A Literature Review.*

11 Liz Walker, Graeme Reid & Morna Cornell, *Waiting to happen: HIV/AIDS in South Africa* (Cape Town: Double Story, 2004).

12 David Arnold, "Cholera and Colonialism in British India," *Past and Present* 113.1 (November 1986): 151, quoted in Harriet Deacon, *Understanding HIV/AIDS Stigma: A Theoretical and Methodological Analysis* (Cape Town: HSRC, 2005): 9.

meanings acquired around important social processes. Theatre can provide sites to name, to speak about that which is left beneath the surface and not spoken about. Unlike more mass-based campaigns such as radio and TV dramas, the invitation to engage physically, emotionally, socially, and in culturally relevant ways with the issues allows applied-theatre practitioners to address the *context-specific* nuances of each group and community. This is exactly what a post-conflict or a post-critical pedagogy calls for.

If theatre has been identified as an effective way to address issues about HIV, how can applied-theatre practices which aim to challenge the status quo and catalyse social and personal transformation work with gendered and patriarchal structures which are fundamental to understanding what is driving HIV infection and mythology? Writers such as Sharon Grady and Kathleen Gallagher argue that applied drama practices are ideally placed to interrupt limiting gender roles and stereotypes.[13] However, some practices, or ideologies that are expressed within these practices, also serve to uphold inequalities either implicitly or explicitly. Louise Bourgault's documentation of some of the plays that young people in a Dramaide programme come up with reveals how patriarchal narratives are played out in how young people dramatize HIV/AIDS:

> They feature young people plagued by sexual advances: young girls the targets of older men [...]. But many of the plays are deeply misogynistic, showing young girls as willing consorts to these men, 'party girls' happy to disobey their parents, go out, and have a good time for the right price.[14]

What is the drama facilitator's ethical role in this context? This is a story created by young people from their own experiences and value-systems. What are the complexities of challenging these value-systems, and how does what happens within the discursive and embodied space of the drama world(s) translate into a wider context?

One of the questions I pose and that remains crucial to understanding how applied theatre can indeed disrupt certain hegemonies and lead to social

---

[13] Sharon Grady, *Drama and Diversity. A Pluralistic Perspective for Educational Drama* (Portsmouth NH: Heinemann, 2000); Kathleen Gallagher, "The Everyday Classroom As Problematic: A Feminist Pedagogy," *Curriculum Inquiry* 30.1 (Spring 2000): 71–81.

[14] Louise Bourgault, *Playing for Life: Performance in Africa in the Age of AIDS* (Durham NC: Carolina Academic Press, 2003): 224.

change is how we navigate the seemingly unique space that is created within the dramatic moment where new identities, stories, and meanings are shaped, and how we negotiate the wider context of, in this case, patriarchy, which is so deeply legitimized and entrenched in the world.

I want to take one moment from my research: This example raised several questions for me as a practitioner. This is a grade 6 group, at a Catholic junior school located in Grahamstown's local township. This is a small group discussion about two characters we had met, an older boy named Siya who was a bit of a player, and a younger girl called Thandi; we were imagining how Thandi might negotiate sex with Siya:

LEARNER GIRL: And Thandi must tell Siya that her body is her marriage if she loses her virginity then she cannot be married and she must be trusted by him.

ALEX: Why is it women are expected to be virgins until married but not men? Do you think that is fair?

LEARNER BOY: It's not fair.

ALEX: Why?

LEARNER BOY: Me, I'm seeing it as fair.

ALEX: It is fair? Why?

LEARNER BOY: Because it's always girls that are always virgins because we as boys are not like girls and we don't have the same body as the girls and so we are different from them.

ALEX: Alright.

LEARNER GIRL: The Bible says you must not have sex before marriage.

ALEX: Is that just for girls?

ALL LEARNERS: No. boys also.

LEARNER GIRL: Boys should hold their horses and wait until married.

ALEX: s that realistic?

LEARNER GIRL: To me, it's not realistic, because some men don't want to wait, they want to have sex.

These young people's received knowledge about how to prevent HIV and to deal with sex is abstinence. But abstinence is not implicitly expected for men. I'm not sure how I disrupt this view, or whether I can. What is the ethical position here? Helen Nicholson defines ethics as "a domain which allows for competing conceptions of the good life" and asks the question that I am now asking as my head races: "what does it mean to act ethically in contexts where there are competing conceptions of the good life?"[15] I am a guest in a Catholic school for whom a true, good life is abstinence. During this discussion about virginity, a young girl starts weeping silently. After the interview she stays behind and I ask her if she is alright. She tells me that her stepfather had 'forced himself on her' and a nurse had told her she was no longer a virgin. She feels dirty, an outsider to her peers, because she has not managed to maintain her virginity, according to a respected medical opinion. The discourse that is shaping her identity as a young woman tells her that she is to blame; she is now soiled. She has not managed to live a 'good' Christian life. I stop thinking about *any* ethical dilemma here. I am no longer the facilitator or the researcher now. I start acting on instinct as I try to tell her another story: you are not to blame.

How do we prepare for these lived experiences that are revealed or disclosed through our drama work? By creating a drama space which deals with distinct binaries such as male vs female, how am I contributing to the repressive myths that Ellsworth critiques? When I analyse the workshop and the catalytic scenes we produced, a male character like Siya is constructed as abusing his charm and power, while Thandi is a young, naive, potential victim. How, the, does this contribute to affirming discourse about abstinence and virginity in our discussion? Sharon Grady poses important questions:

> How do teachers inadvertently contribute to gender role stereotyping in their drama work? How do limiting assumptions about gender roles affect identity formation? How can drama teachers and theatre for youth practitioners actively avoid these traps as they structure dramatic situations?[16]

How does, or can, the relationship between art, life, the social, and the artistic work to make a difference? I return to Neelands' perspectives on how theatre might mediate art and life. Drawing on the philosopher Walter Benjamin, he argues that "a state of emergency is also a state of necessary *emergence*."[17] HIV and the gender inequalities that drive it are a state of emergency, and demand the emergence of alternative gendered identities. By reducing the

---

[15] Helen Nicholson, *Drama: The Gift of Theatre* (Basingstoke: Palgrave Macmillan, 2005): 157.

[16] Sharon Grady, *Drama and Diversity*, 80.

[17] Neelands, "Miracles are happening," 52.

complexities of power relationships to the 'oppressor' and 'the oppressed', I, like many other theatre practitioners who try to address one of the most urgent social issues of our time, have fallen into the trap of showing only one version of how things *are*. Part of my disillusionment is in my own limited approaches. Why do we show the way the world is, not what it might be becoming? Jansen's proposal for a post-conflict pedagogy is vital. Although he is talking about issues of race here, extrapolations to other 'divisions' such as gender can also be made:

> A post-conflict pedagogy is founded on hope. It does not get lost within a circularity of oppression talk where whites retell stories of 'them' as being less and blacks retell stories of 'us' as being harmed. It is strongly against any sense of victimhood, for this traps [us] in an endlessly downward spiral of defeat. This kind of critical pedagogy recognizes the power and the pain at play in school and society, and their effects on young people, and asks "*how*" things could be better [...]. Hope starts by asking that same question within the pedagogical situation: *"how do I move towards'* in order to relocate to a safer and more secure place, with others.[18]

A challenge for me as a practitioner and researcher is how to engage audiences and participants to construct these *becomings*, these emergences, rather than always focusing on the emergency. How do I construct dramatic spaces that enable us to move towards?

WORKS CITED

Arnold, David. "Cholera and Colonialism in British India," *Past and Present* 113.1 (November 1986): 118–51.

Bourgault, Louise. *Playing for Life: Performance in Africa in the Age of AIDS* (Durham NC: Carolina Academic Press, 2003).

Deacon, Harriet. *Understanding HIV/AIDS Stigma: A Theoretical and Methodological Analysis* (Cape Town: HSRC, 2005).

Ellsworth, Elizabeth. "Why Doesn't This Feel Empowering? Working Through the Repressive Myths of Critical Pedagogy," *Harvard Educational Review* 59.3 (August 1989): 297–324.

Gallagher, Kathleen. "The Everyday Classroom As Problematic: A Feminist Pedagogy," *Curriculum Inquiry* 30.1 (Spring 2000): 71–81.

[18] Jansen, "On the Clash of Martyrological Memories," 154–55.

Grady, Sharon. *Drama and Diversity. A Pluralistic Perspective for Educational Drama* (Portsmouth NH: Heinemann, 2000).

——. "Feminist methodology," in *Research Methodologies for Drama Education*, ed. Judith Ackroyd (Stoke-on-Trent: Trentham, 2006): 81–110.

Jansen, Jonathan D. "On the Clash of Martyrological Memories," *Perspectives in Education* 27.2 (June 2009): 147–57.

Kistner, Ulrike. *Gender-Based Violence and HIV/AIDS in South Africa: A Literature Review* (Johannesburg: CADRE, 2003).

Neelands, Jonothan. "Miracles are happening: beyond the rhetoric of transformation in the Western traditions of drama education," *RiDE: Research in Drama Education* 9.1 (2004): 47–56.

Nicholson, Helen. *Drama: The Gift of Theatre* (Basingstoke: Palgrave Macmillan, 2005).

Walker, Liz, Graeme Reid & Morna Cornell. *Waiting to Happen: HIV/AIDS in South Africa* (Cape Town: Double Story, 2004).

⌘

GALIA BONEH

This Is My Story

A Model for Creating Performance Engaging Artists and People Living with HIV/AIDS

AIDS ACTIVISTS AND SCHOLARS have long been calling for inclusion of People Living with HIV/AIDS (PLWHA) in HIV education and advocacy. In this essay I present a novel model for creating performance through the collaboration of PLWHA and professional and/or student artists. The model was developed in Ghana, together with the performing artist Iddi Saaka, as part of my doctoral dissertation in Culture and Performance, under the auspices of the Center for Art | Global Health at the University of California, Los Angeles.

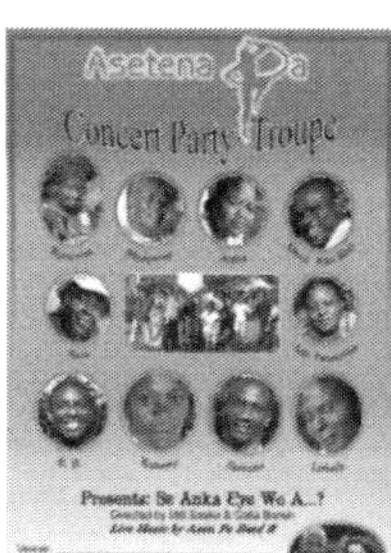
Asetena Pa
Concert Party Troupe

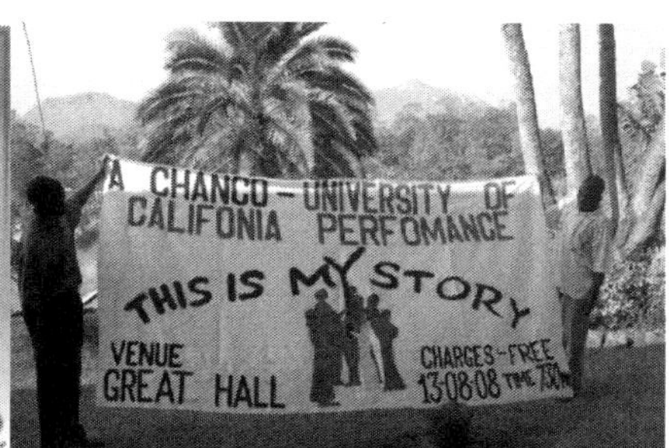
A CHANCO – UNIVERSITY OF CALIFONIA PERFOMANCE
THIS IS MY STORY
VENUE
GREAT HALL
CHARGES-FREE
13.08.08

Figure 1: "Se Anka Eye Wo a…"; Figure 2: "This Is My Story"

The model was developed through the Asetena pa Project which took place in Ghana in 2006. The project engaged five PLWHA and five famous Concert

Party[1] actors. The group underwent an intensive two-week process culminating in the creation of a concert party titled, in the local language of Twi, "Se Anka Eye Wo a..." ('If it were you....'), which then toured eleven towns across Ghana.

In 2008 the model was applied again through the CHANCO-UCLA HIV/AIDS Performance Project which took place in Chancellor College of the University of Malawi. The project engaged fourteen Chancellor College drama students, six local PLWHA actors, and three University of California students, in a more spread-out five-week process that culminated in the creation of a performance titled 'This Is My Story'. The performance was staged at Chancellor College at a nearby teacher's training college campus.

The active engagement of PLWHA in the creative process and performance has several benefits. First, the input of people who have had first-hand experience of the medical, social, cultural, economic, and political challenges of HIV/AIDS can assist in creating deep understanding of these issues. PLWHA bring real stories and rich material for creation that is grounded in reality. Secondly, performance on the topic of HIV/AIDS will necessarily include some form of representation of PLWHA, and it is only right that PLWHA take part in shaping that representation. Third, the experience is empowering for the participating PLWHA and for PLWHA among the audiences, and their active participation and presence on stage shatters stereotypes of PLWHA as passive and weak. Finally, the very collaboration of people with HIV and people who do not have HIV, seeing them together on stage touching, embracing, joking, singing, and acting together, sends out a clear and loud message of acceptance.

Alongside the PLWHA, the model requires the participation of people who have talent and experience in performance of local artforms and who are socially and culturally affiliated with the target audiences. This is to ensure that the production is of high quality and is grounded in the local culture. These can be professional performing artists or university students majoring in performance-art forms. In Ghana, the performance was intended for the general public, and therefore the chosen performance form was the popular Concert Party. In Malawi, the target audience was university students, who tend to belong to the urban, modern elite; thus, the relevant artistic form, and the one the students were most comfortable with, was conventional theatre.

---

[1] Concert Party is a popular Ghanaian performance form that includes music, comedy, and drama.

Four Principles

The working model of the project was guided by four basic principles, described briefly below:

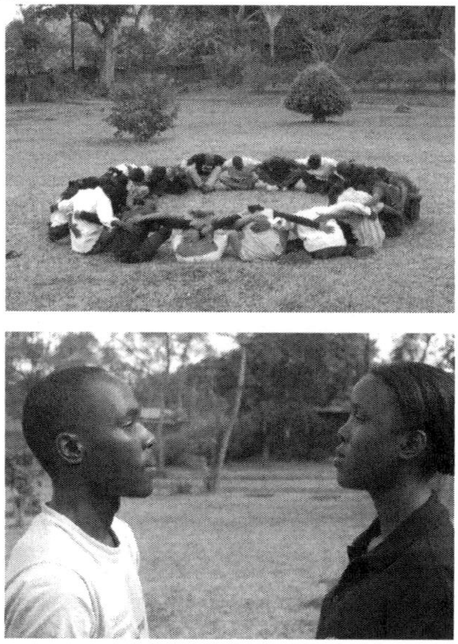

Figures 3 and 4: Process–Product Balance

The more conventional model of creating art for HIV education is top-down: Funding agencies decide on the message and hire the artists to use their skills and talent to deliver the message. The voice they represent is that of the agency who hired them; there is no place for their own voices. In process-oriented work, artists are asked to engage intellectually and emotionally in analysing the social problem, and through such engagement explore and form their own voices. And yet, the work does result in a performance, unlike work that is entirely process-oriented and does not necessarily reach the stage. The time spent on the project is divided equally between process-oriented work (creating intimacy in the group, sharing of personal stories, exploration of issues, forming of voices) and product-oriented work (casting, rehearsals, production).

It should be noted that the result is not a perfect, scripted, and well-rehearsed performance, but one that is largely based on improvisation, simple setting and costume design, and in general not exhibiting high production values.

Rather, it is more intimate, based on the interaction and human qualities of the participants.

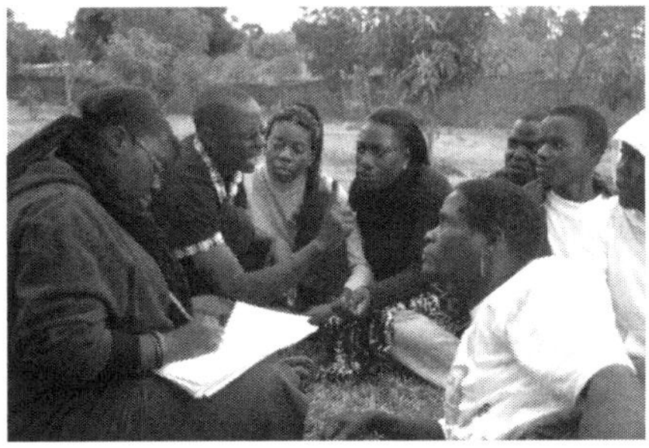

Figure 5: From Messaging to Critical Thinking

'Persuasive communication' or 'messaging' carries the risk of being condescending, and over-simplifying the challenges it seeks to address. Structural problems such as poverty, gender inequality, and lack of infrastructure are still ignored in campaigns, which continue to offer slogan solutions that are irrelevant to people's lives.

Rather than assuming that people will do as we tell them, in this model we propose to shift our way of thinking away from 'messaging' and instead concentrate our efforts on stimulating a lively dialogue and an active response grounded in reality: in other words, to trigger a participatory process of critical thinking.

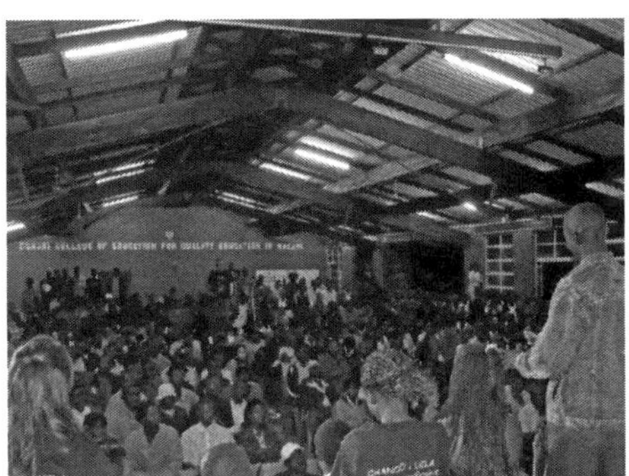

Figure 6: Targeting the Community

In her book *Letting Them Die*, Catherine Campbell draws attention to the fact that the HIV/AIDS epidemic has largely been analysed at the micro-social and macro-social levels. The micro-social level has to do with properties of the individual, such as cognitive processes, attitudes, sense of personal vulnerability, and perceived social norms. The macro-social level focuses on the ways in which poverty, gender inequality, and global capitalism shape the contexts in which the epidemic flourishes. She writes: "However, little attention has been paid to the way in which these micro and macro factors interact at the local community level."[2] She further explains:

> Local communities often form the contexts within which people negotiate their social and sexual lives and identities [...]. They equally often play a key role in enabling or restraining people from taking control over their health.[3]

Live performance is attended by several members of the community, making it a shared experience. It joins the range of festivals, weddings, funerals, and other social and cultural occasions where communal norms and values are formed and revisited. Through the use of local performance forms, expressions, cultural icons, and shared heritage, new discourses are organically introduced into the ongoing process of change, redefinition, and revisiting of the groups' identity and values. The shared experience also generates discussion in the community hours, days and even weeks after the performance.

Specifically regarding HIV/AIDS and sexual behaviour, a live performance attended by both sexes can serve as an opening for vitally important intimate discussions that are difficult to initiate in other ways. The performance and a following question-and-answer session can spur further discussions in the community.

From Compassion to Empowerment

Perhaps in an attempt to correct the damage caused by the scare campaigns of the early 1980s and 1990s, in recent years the concept of showing compassion to PLWHA has been advocated in campaigns worldwide. While compassion appears to be a positive sentiment to evoke, a closer look may question this assumption. Let us consider the following images of billboards that were photographed in Ghana, West Africa, in 2007:

---

[2] Catherine Campbell, *Letting Them Die: Why HIV Prevention Programs Fail* (Bloomington: Indiana UP, 2003): 2.

[3] Campbell, *Letting Them Die*, 3.

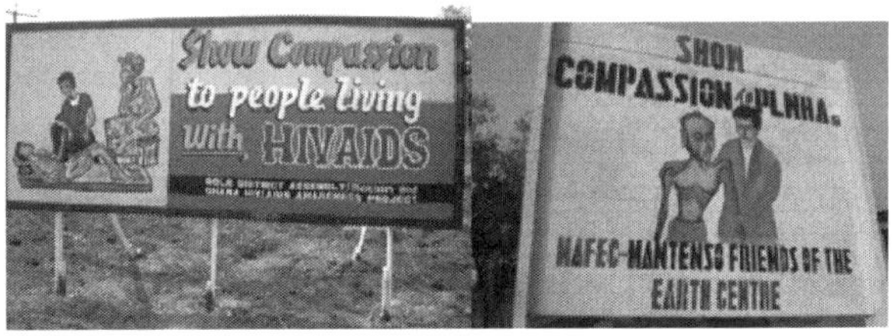
Show Compassion
to people living
with HIV/AIDS
SHOW
COMPASSION to PLWHA.
MAFEC-MANTENSO FRIENDS OF THE
EARTH CENTRE

Figures 7 and 8: Victimhood and Compassion

In both images, the person living with HIV/AIDS still appears as a victim, as customary in earlier portrayals of PLWHA. He still appears to be dying and still shows signs of weakness and powerlessness. In both images, the people showing compassion are situated higher than the PLWHA, looking down at him or her.

The concept of compassion sets in stone the uneven dynamic in which the receiver of compassion is rendered powerless, needy of mercy or pity, and dependent on the goodwill of the giver of compassion, who in effect holds the power. This observation leads us to ask: Is it compassion that PLWHA need from their families, general public, and government – or do they need the power to exercise their own human rights, demand fair and equal treatment, and not be dependent on the goodwill of others? Does the concept of compassion not fuel the cycle of 'victimhood', and if so, what alternative concept would be both more inspiring and liberating, and more useful in countering the spread of the epidemic?

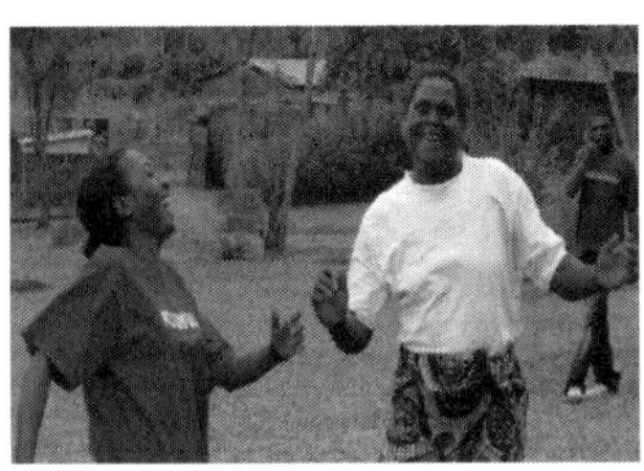

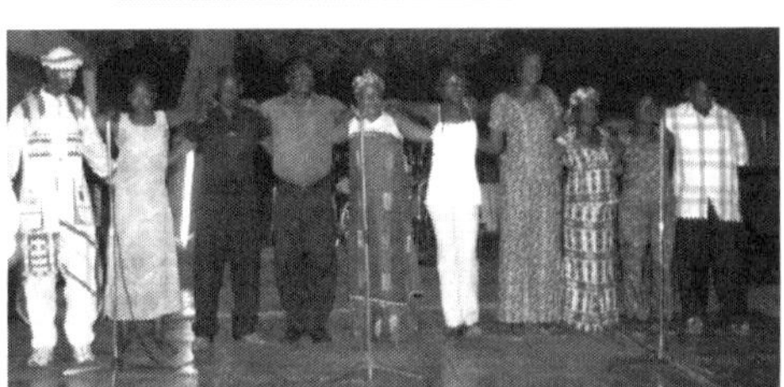

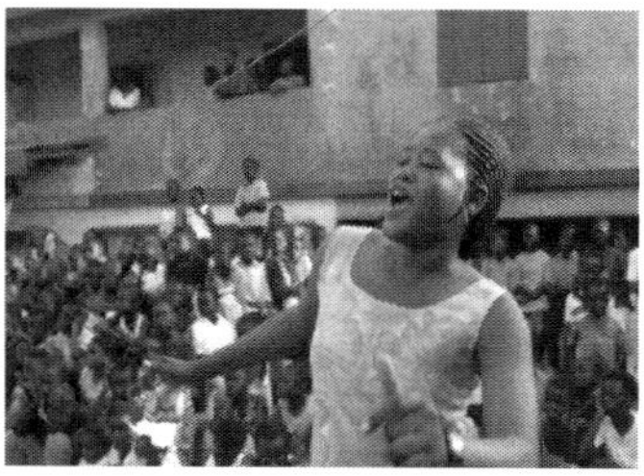

Figures 9, 10, and 11: Vitality in Performance

Live performance in which performing PLWHA are vocal, confident – singing, dancing, acting – *alive* – can be a powerful and transformative image that may alter the deeply engrained images of PLWHA as passive victims, sick, dying, etc. Moreover, if the performing PLWHA undergo a process of personal empowerment during the production, the content of their messages, and even their body language, will enhance the general movement from compassion to empowerment. More profound than what they say is the image of them, speaking up.

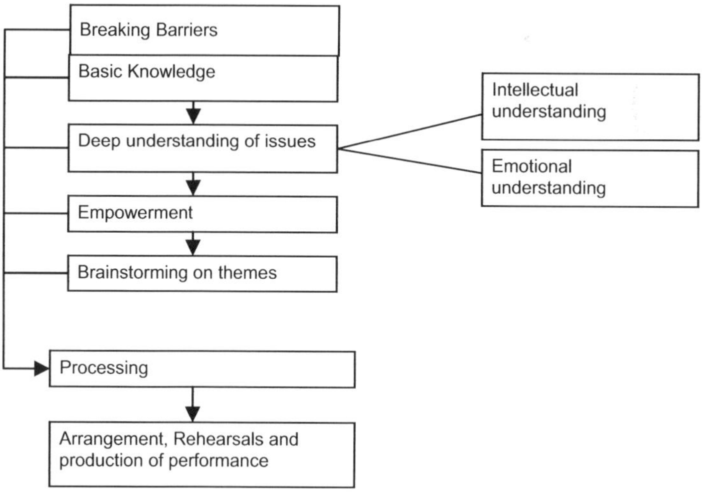

Figure 12: From Breaking Barriers to Performance

Empowered PLWHA will not only assist themselves and others like them to live fuller, happier lives, but will also assist in countering the epidemic. The notion that people can live full lives with HIV/AIDS can give courage to others to test themselves for HIV, and seek treatment if necessary. If their empowerment leads to a shift in the attitudes of the general public towards PLWHA, it is possible that revealing one's HIV positive status to one's partner will become easier and more widespread, thereby preventing future infections. An empowered PLWHA can generate discussion, educate, and share personal experience that can be useful in encouraging preventive behaviour. Finally, collective empowerment of PLWHA can create a functional network and lobby that may bring about improved facilities, access to treatment, legislation, and other structural changes.

The Working Model

The four principles noted above are translated into practice through the following working model. After selecting the participants (artists/students and PLWHA), and meeting with each group separately to address any anxieties they had, the participants undergo an intensive training of approximately 100 hours. Ideally, the group would work six to eight hours a day for two to three weeks. In the CHANCO-UCLA Performance Project, the 100 hours were spread across five weeks, since the students were not available to engage in the project full-time. The structure of the workshop is as follows:

Breaking barriers: The first couple days of the workshop are devoted solely to getting to know one another, creating one group out of the two groups that came together for the project, and creating an atmosphere of trust. This is done through music, movement, and theatre games. Throughout the workshop, each day opens with a few of these exercises, in order to maintain the special atmosphere that has been created throughout the whole workshop.

Basic knowledge: In order to avoid misinformation and inaccuracy in the performance, it is important to get the basic facts right. This is particularly important, as audiences tend to view performers as experts on the topic and often approach them with questions after the show. Information sessions are delivered in the next phase of the workshop by a professional counselor or medical doctor who specializes in HIV/AIDS.

Deep understanding of issues: Deep understanding, both intellectually and emotionally, of the challenges surrounding HIV/AIDS is achieved by three major activities, which take place during the third phase of the workshop: sharing of personal stories; holding debates on related topics; and theatre exercises that stimulate discussion and understanding of the complexities of reality.

Empowerment: Empowerment of the participants is achieved throughout the whole process, especially through the relationships formed in the group, and culminating with their experience on stage. However, the fourth phase of the creative process is devoted specifically to exercises that explore possibilities and sources of power within oppressive situations.

Brainstorming on themes: The activities noted above take approximately fifty hours (half of the workshop's duration). After establishing intimacy, discussing, listening, gaining understanding, insights and ideas, brainstorming sessions are held on the issues that have come up and seem relevant and important to treat in the performance. At first we list every idea that was suggested, and then vote to choose one major topic, recognizing that some of the other issues can be represented as sub-topics.

Processing: After selecting the theme, we split up into two groups, with each group generating a general storyline based on the material accumulated in the course of the workshop. The directors then use the theme and the suggested storylines as a guide, and write a unified storyline which they then present back to the group. Adjustments are made after receiving feedback from the group.

Arrangement, rehearsals and production of Performance: Casting is done through auditions, but it is the participants, not the directors, who (through secret ballot) choose the actors for each role. All participants are given a role in the play. After assigning roles, we arrange each scene, rehearse, add costumes and props, etc.

The work of production is also done by the participants: they divide into groups and each group is in charge of a different aspect of production such as set design, costumes and props, and advertisement.

Performance: In both projects, at the end of the performance there is a shift from the fiction of the play to real life: The performance ends with the actors introducing themselves as real people: Their names, whether they are HIV-positive or -negative (if positive – how many years they have been living with HIV), and a brief statement about themselves. The statements are voluntary (made only by performers who wish to make them) and are written by the performers themselves. For audiences, this is the moment at which everything becomes real – it is a moment of surprise, transformation, reflection – and the beginning of several discussions to come – right after the performance and days and weeks to follow. Following each performance, a question-and-answer session is held to initiate these conversations.

The important feature of the model is that the product is a reflection of the process. The relationships between the participants are reflected on stage; the complexity of reality we discover during the first phases of the creative process is reflected in the content of the performance; and the spirit of group work is reflected in all aspects of the production.

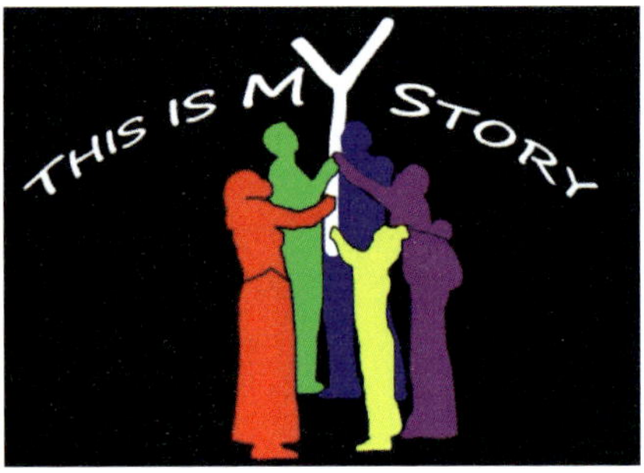

Figure 13: This Is My Story

Synopsis of *This Is My Story*

— Created by the CHANCO-UCLA Performance Project, Zomba, Malawi 2008

This Is My Story is a story of a final-year female university student, Chisomo, who is madly in love with her boyfriend Kumbu. Kumbu, well aware of Chisomo's blind love, has other girlfriends on the side. Although his friends help him keep his actions secret, Chisomo suspects that something is going on, and this causes her to lose concentration on her studies, and her grades to plunge. When she receives her test results, she realizes the impact this could have on her life, and she approaches her professors, asking for a chance to re-write. One of her instructors, Mr. Tipicos, a married man and father of two (with the third on its way), abuses his power, and asks that she date him in exchange for a "second chance." Chisomo, at first angry at the proposal, eventually feels she has no choice but to agree if she wishes to pass the exams and graduate.

Time goes by; Mr, Tipico's baby is born, but is often sick. His wife returns from the hospital furious: she has found out she and the baby are HIV-positive. She decides to leave him. Mr. Tipico's sinks into depression, and word about what has happened reaches the students. When Chisomo hears the rumours she is scared and confused. She visits her aunt, who encourages her to get tested and promises her support. Chisomo tests HIV-positive. With her aunt's support and personal strength she manages to go on with her life, keeping her secret to herself, immersing herself in her studies.

As she becomes withdrawn, the tables turn and her boyfriend Kumbu grows more in love with her, constantly courting her and begging for her forgiveness for his wrongdoing. Chisomo rejects his approaches, but the more she refuses, the keener he becomes on getting her back. Eventually she agrees to take him back. In the meantime, Mr. Tipicos, full of remorse, approaches the elders in his family, asking that they beg his wife, on his behalf, to come back.

In her room, Chisomo tries to imagine how Kumbu would react if she were to tell him of her HIV status. After playing through different versions in her mind, she decides that she cannot tell him. The next time he comes over is their first romantic encounter since they got back together. When things begin to heat up, Chisomo asks that he use a condom. Kumbu dismisses her request, but when she insists, he gets offended and angry. He interprets her insistence as lack of trust in him, or lack of trust in herself. As he walks away she shouts "I am just trying to protect you!"

In the final scene, during their graduation, Mrs. Tipicos returns, but the scene freezes before we see her encounter with her husband. Kumbu approaches Chisomo, but the scene freezes before we hear what he says. Instead, the singers in the group raise the theme song "I-Ndiyo Kani Yanga" (Chichewa for 'This is my story – what is yours?') and, one by one, the PLWHA in the group, as well as some of the students, touch the character they identify most with (causing that character to sit down) and come forward, addressing the audience: 'My name is so and so. This is my story because…..'

The statements made were written by the PLWHA and the students who volunteered to speak. Below are some examples:

> *Subira:* This is my story because like many women, I too have been affected by HIV. My name is Subira. I have been living with HIV for 4 years. I was a faithful wife, but 3 years into marriage I got sick.

After tests were done I was found HIV-positive. When I confronted my husband I had discovered that he had deliberately infected me. I had trusted him when he told me he had tested negative before we got married. Some may call this stupidity, but those who have been in love know how trust issues work.

It broke my heart and almost broke my spirit but after a while, I reached deep inside me and drew on my inner strength. I took control of my life against all odds. I forgave and with forgiveness came great power to live my life to the full. Knowing my status didn't kill me, it only made me stronger.

Natalia: My name is Natalia and I am a 4th year student. This is also my story because my boyfriend broke up with me because I suggested we use a condom.

Levison: My name is Levison. I have been living with HIV for a year. This is my story because I am like Kumbu's girlfriend in the play. When I found out I was HIV positive, I tried to protect my wife by using condoms but she has been refusing despite the fact that she is negative.

Because of her refusal, I decided that I was not going to put her life at risk by letting her have her way knowing it can destroy her life. I have told her that the only way she can protect herself is by using a condom.

She has continued to refuse and I have made a decision that it is better to divorce her than put her life at risk.

Simunye: My name is Simunye. I am a third-year. This is also my story because I once had a boyfriend who cheated on me.

Leonard: This is also my story because I have been living with HIV for five years. My story is similar to Professor Tipico's in the play who loved girls and women. I was also a womanizer in my youth, up to the time I got married.

When I got married and a few years had passed, in 2003 my wife started getting sick often as well as our child. We decided to go for testing. Both my wife and I were found positive; so was the child. After a year, both my wife and child had died.

I was devastated, because I knew I was responsible for their deaths. Even now it still hurts me.

In 2006 I married another wife who has the same status as me. We are living happily and depend on each other always using condoms in our family.

> I am also a member of Reach Trust Organization where I lead 178 HIV-positive people.

After nine such statements, one by one all the other participants come to the front of the stage, saying 'this is my story because…', each person telling how they personally connect to the story, forming a line of all participants facing the audience speaking over one another. The last person to join the line says 'This is my story because...' and all together the group responds: 'This is Our Story!'; Lights Out.

Impact

Both projects (in Ghana and in Malawi) were evaluated for their impact on the participants and audiences. In Ghana, four focus groups separated by sex and age were conducted following four of the performances (total of sixteen focus groups). Data was analysed and presented in my PhD dissertation. In Malawi, UCLA PGH conducted 74 semi-structured interviews in June 2009, among largely Chancellor College students, to assess the impact of the *This Is My Story* project one year after the performance. The questionnaires were designed a) to determine if there was a greater understanding among Chancellor College students of the benefits and barriers to HIV prevention and treatment, and b) to evaluate whether attitudes and/or forms of behaviour changed in terms of the prevention of HIV and reduction in stigma as a result of the project. Data is currently being analysed and will be published in the near future.

Impact on participants

Both projects proved to be life-changing experiences for all participants. Below are selected observations by some of the participants in the CHANCO-UCLA Performance Project in Malawi:

> Through my engagement with the CHANCO-UCLA project I have been empowered. Because of this project, for the first time in my life I went for VCT so as to know my status. I enjoyed performing, therefore to me both the process and product of this performance project has been enriching.
> — Sylvester Chapotera

> This whole process has been a life changing experience for me. The discussions gave me insight as to what young people think, the challenges they face, how they cope with pressure from society and their

> peers. But it was also a learning experience because when you are affected by HIV you sometimes forget that there are people out there who may not realize how serious the epidemic is. It was also an opportunity to share our stories, that some may take lessons that may save their lives and protect their futures. I am happy to say I believe we have achieved our goal
> — Subira Msumba.

> The project was very good because it has shown me how courageous and strong-hearted we people living with HIV are. The other thing that touched me was the bonds that were formed between people living with HIV and the students and directors. There was no discrimination.
> — Medson Leonard Lenzo

> The project has really changed my life. The stories that were told made me think about my own life. I had this inner fear about HIV/AIDS and now I know so much about it and with the knowledge I have gained from this group I will be able to reach out to others and change their lives just as it did change mine. Others are still in denial as they have not come into contact with PLWHA. Words cannot express what a big difference it has brought to my life
> — Ghawubupi Angela Mwabungulu

> This project was a great experience because I made new friends, most of whom have had a great impact on my life, especially the PLWHA. For example, when I decide to go for VCT, trust me, I will not call my dad, mom, aunt or anyone else. I will Subira because she has become a great role model in my life.
> — Natalia Ngosiani Govati

As evident in the above quotations, the most meaningful aspect of the project was the intimate interaction between the students and the PLWHA. This interaction proved to be empowering and inspiring for both.

Impact on audiences

One of the themes assessed in the focus groups conducted in Ghana was audience response to the involvement of PLWHA in the production. The initial reaction of respondents in the majority of the focus groups was controversy over whether the testimonies were true. The significance of the controversy lies in the implications of believing the testimonies were true and a reading of the performance as a display of reality and not mere fiction. One of the notable emotional reactions was fear, due to the realization that there may not be any visible signs to indicate that a person is infected with HIV, and therefore one cannot protect him- or herself merely by associating with healthy-looking people, as evident in the following passage:

> Yesterday what made me sad when I stood there watching the performance was, all the people [women] who were performing were very beautiful. If I had the chance I would have approached them [to court them]. But at the end when they came out and said I have this and I have that, my legs were no longer on the floor.[4]

At the same time, many respondents reacted with feelings of happiness and hope derived from the image of PLWHA as healthy and strong individuals, the courageous act of public disclosure, and the friendly interaction between the PLWHA and the professional actors.

> I don't know how to describe how I felt when they said they were positive because most people try to hide this sickness from the general public and they were so bold to come out to the public and say that, it was really marvelous.[5]

> It pleased me so much that they were able to open their hearts to tell us they have it. For my idea was that if one has AIDS he dies within a few months, or grows lean, but I saw that some of them were even fatter than those without AIDS! [6]

The active participation of PLWHA in the production also served as proof to the various messages that were transmitted in the performance: Information regarding treatment was proven true through the healthy looking bodies and vitality of the performers; Information regarding modes of transmission, and the safety in ordinary interaction with PLWHA, was proven through the interaction of actors and PLWHA.

> I was so happy because though some were positive and some were not yet they all came together to act the play and related very well. This means that we can also do things together with our own folks who are positive.[7]

The participation of the PLWHA also contributed to shifts in attitudes towards PLWHA and towards the concept of disclosure as a result of the performance.

---

[4] Man, Damongo, 30 November 2006.

[5] Woman, Bamboi, 28 November 2006.

[6] Man, Bole, 1 December 2006.

[7] Man, Bamboi, 28 November 2006.

Conclusion

The active participation of PLWHA in the creative process and performance is not only an empowering experience for performers but also one that triggers lively public discourse that questions many of the previously held assumptions and stereotypes in the community. The working model hereby presented guides the collaborative creation by PLWHA and professional/student performing artists, through an intensive and deep process that is grounded in reality and the local culture.

WORK CITED

Campbell, Catherine. *Letting Them Die: Why HIV Prevention Programs Fail* (Bloomington: Indiana UP, 2003).

For more information, please visit www.makeartstopaids.org or email galiaboneh@gmail.com

⌘

Kennedy Chinyowa

A Poetic of Contradictions?

HIV/AIDS Interventions at the Crossroads of Localization and Globalization

Introduction

The emergence of applied-theatre practice in African contexts, where it is generally known as popular theatre, occurred in response to the apparent shortcomings of the discourse of modern economic development. Up to the mid-1970s, development as a process of bettering the lives of disadvantaged people had largely been premised on externally driven intervention models. However, by the time of the United Nations Decade for Cultural Development (1988–97), it became increasingly evident that the economic principles informing modern economic development had overlooked the significance of cultural factors in the so-called Third World. Modern scientific and technological progress had not been accompanied by the much desired peace, prosperity, and security but by increasing poverty, hunger, malnutrition, disease, crime, and violence. It therefore comes as no surprise that local, national, and international development agencies are now searching for development alternatives that are grounded in the lived experiences of local communities – what UNESCO has described as the "cultural dimension of development."[1]

As a function of the cultural-development paradigm, applied-theatre practice appears to have found itself 'standing' at the crossroads of both economic

---

[1] UNESCO, *The Cultural Dimension of Development: Towards a Practical Approach* (Paris: UNESCO, 1995).

and cultural-development discourses. While the more globalized economic-development paradigm continues to be what Arturo Escobar calls "a top-down, ethnocentric and technocratic approach which treats people and cultures as abstract concepts, statistical figures to be moved up and down in the chart of progress,"[2] the more localized cultural-development paradigm insists on deriving its inspiration from the target communities' aesthetic frames of reference. The latter insists on treating people not as "statistical figures" but as subjects who can participate in the making of their own history.

This essay argues that applied theatre is more of a political activity, surrounded by a bundle of contradictions. It is concerned with interventions that attempt to bring change in relations of power among individuals and within communities. The participants who engage in it – practitioners (or facilitators) and beneficiaries – are implicated in a political process that resonates with tensions arising from questions of agency, representation, authority, and ownership. Such politics has a far-reaching influence on the aesthetics (or poetics) of the work (process), the outcomes of the work (product), and its impact on the target audience. Any meaningful evaluation of applied-theatre practice therefore needs to consider the negative contradictions surrounding the work. For instance, while the facilitator may be driven by the desire to enable the community to set its own local agenda on development, that agenda often clashes with the global agenda of the funding agency or, at times, with the ambiguous ideology of the facilitator.

If practitioners were transparent about their intentions, about the 'baggage' they bring into their work, it could have been possible to avoid the tensions that seem to characterize the local aspirations of target communities and the global desires of practitioners. But because practitioners often tend to manipulate the process to suit their ideological ends, the practice of applied theatre appears to have remained at the crossroads in terms of both process and product. There are questions that still remain unanswered, such as: For whom are the projects meant? Whose reality counts? Who counts that reality? How is that reality counted? Using examples drawn from selected HIV/AIDS interventions, this essay focuses on the aesthetic contradictions that have arisen from the polarity between localization and globalization. In particular, the essay examines three selected aesthetic categories – folk media, participation,

---

[2] Arturo Escobar, *Encountering Development: The Making and Unmaking of the Third World* (Princeton NJ: Princeton UP, 1995): 44.

and syncretism – that have informed applied-theatre interventions on HIV/AIDS and posits possibilities based on the principles of critical pedagogy.[3]

Folk Media

Folk media have been described as the vehicle by which the common people, such as peasants and workers, communicate their ideas, values, and beliefs.[4] The centrality of folk media as an aesthetic in development communication became prominent during the shift from the modern-development paradigm to "the cultural dimension of development."[5] However, as Nici Nelson and Susan Wright[6] have argued, the shift towards the discourse of the marginalized, whom they call "the primary stakeholders," has been more *instrumental* than *transformational*. More often than not, communities are led into participating in workshops using 'folk' songs, dances, poems, and stories that have already been planned for them. Nelson and Wright assert that it is instrumental to *get* people to take part in workshops, and transformative when such people have power to decide on their own priorities. Robert Chambers sums it up when he says the instrumental paradigm means that 'they' (local people) participate in 'our' project as opposed to the transformational in which 'we' participate in 'their' project.[7]

Thus, when folk media are instrumental, communities have less control over the process that is supposed to empower them. For instance, in a report

---

[3] Peter McLaren, *Critical Pedagogy and Predatory Culture* (New York & London: Routledge, 1995); Henry Giroux, *Border Crossings: Cultural Workers and the Politics of Education* (New York & London: Routledge, 1992); Antonia Darder, Marta Baltodano & Rodolfo Torres, ed. *Critical Pedagogy Reader* (London & New York: RoutledgeFalmer, 2003).

[4] James L. Ng'ombe, "The Communication Model and Folk Media in Development," in *Sustainable Development Dimensions*. Food and Agricultural Organisation (FAO) (2000), http://www.fao.org/sd/CDdirect/CDan0029.htm)

[5] UNESCO, *The Cultural Dimension of Development.*

[6] Nici Nelson & Susan Wright, "Participation and Power," in *Power and Participatory Development: Theory and Practice*, ed. Nelson & Wright (London: Intermediate Technology, 1995): 1–18.

[7] Robert Chambers, "Paradigm shifts and the practice of participatory research and development," in *Power and Participatory Development: Theory and Practice*, ed. Nici Nelson & Susan Wright (London: Intermediate Technology, 1995): 30.

on a workshop that was carried out in Malawi by the Food and Agricultural Organisation's (FAO) Communication for Development Group to explore how folk media was used by the people in order to facilitate the process of development, it was noted that most external intervention programmes were replete with examples of well-meaning efforts that end up frustrated by a lack of appreciation of local communication systems.[8] The group cited one instance where puppetry, such as *nyau* masks, was used among the Chewa people, whose culture associates puppetry with the world of animals and spirits. By implication, the development effort became a contradiction in terms because it attempted to explain 'rational' behaviour through 'irrational' means,[9] at least in the eyes of the local people.

Michael Balfour points out that applied theatre suffers from what he calls the crisis of aesthetic engagement.[10] Quite often, when practitioners intervene in local communities, they appear as cultural missionaries acting on behalf of donors. Rather than allowing communities to set their own agenda, practitioners tend to impose ideological values derived from their funders. In such instances, it is not the 'oppressed' or 'subalterns' who need their consciousness to be raised but the practitioners, who are unaware of their contradictory position as emissaries of global ideologies that may be at odds with local aspirations. The option is for practitioners to acknowledge the validity of indigenous ways of knowing such as folk media. As Syed Jamil Ahmed has argued, in the process of wanting to make the subaltern's voice heard, practitioners often misconstrue such voices in their own image. Instead, subaltern silence can be regarded as a form of subtle resistance against dominant or oppressive forces.[11]

---

[8] Philippe van der Stichele, "Folk and traditional media for rural development: a workshop held in Malawi," in *Sustainable Development Dimensions* (Food and Agricultural Organisation (FAO), 2000), http://www.fao.org/sd/CDdirect/CDan0029.htm (accessed 28 July 2011).

[9] Christopher Kamlongera, *Theatre for Development in Africa with Case Studies from Malawi and Zambia* (Bonn: German Foundation for International Development, 1988).

[10] Michael Balfour, "The politics of intention: looking for a theatre of little changes," *RiDE: Research in Drama Education* 14.3 (August 2009): 354.

[11] Syed Jamil Ahmed, "Examining interventionist theatre in a multi-axial world of transience: An essay in refusal," in *Drama as Social Intervention*, ed. Michael Balfour & John W. Somers (Concord, Ontario: Captus University Publications, 2006): 51–52.

Perhaps folk media best illustrate how subalterns can express themselves in their own way. This is evident from the use of folk media in HIV/AIDS interventions by Amakhosi Theatre, a leading popular-theatre organization based in Bulawayo, Zimbabwe. In their HIV/AIDS play entitled *Vikela* (protect yourself), the group opens with a Ndebele folk dance called *isitshikitsha* accompanied by a song. The female dancers, clad in traditional *indlukula* costume made from animal skin kilts and headgear, adopt a call-and-response technique for the song by calling out:

> Who spread HIV/AIDS *lapa ekhaya* (here at home)?
> You spread HIV/AIDS *lapa ekhaya!*
> Who? Me?
> Yes! You! (extract from *Vikela* video).

The opening song-and-dance movement can be regarded as a way of showing how people express their fear of HIV/AIDS by blaming others. More specifically, the folk dance serves as an incriminating metaphor for those who want to stigmatize people with HIV/AIDS. Such folk media function as an aesthetic device by which community-theatre practitioners can frame their performances by using local performance idioms.

Similarly, Lynn Dalrymple, the co-founder of the Drama in AIDS Education (DramAidE) organization based in Durban, South Africa, regards folk media as a cultural frame of reference for most local community activities.[12] Dalrymple[13] has written extensively on how folk media can be used to explore people's beliefs, attitudes, and practices. For instance, in their HIV/AIDS play entitled *See You at 7*,[14] DramAidE attempts to integrate ritual

---

[12] Lynn Dalrymple, *A Drama Approach to AIDS Education: A Report on an AIDS and Lifestyles Education Project Undertaken in a Rural School in Zululand* (Kwa Dlangezwa: University of Zululand, 1992).

[13] Dalrymple, *A Drama Approach to AIDS Education*; "Is DramAidE Making a Difference?" in *Monitoring and Evaluation Handbook* (KwaDlangezwa: University of Zululand, 1995); "The DramAidE Project," in *Drama, Culture and Empowerment: The IDEA Dialogues*, ed. John O'Toole & Kate Donelan (Brisbane: IDEA Publications, 1996): 33–36; "DramAidE: An evaluation of interactive drama and theatre for HIV/AIDS education in South Africa," in *Drama as Social Intervention*, ed. Michael Balfour & John W. Somers (Concord, Ontario: Captus University Publications, 2006): 195–206.

[14] Lynn Dalrymple & Paul Botha, *A Facilitator's Guide to See You at 7* (Kwa Dlangezwa: Atlas Printers, 2001).

structure as a processual element for the forum theatre intervention. The DramAidE team simply creates a platform for dramatic action, and invites the target audience to take over the process using their own performance idioms. For taboo subjects associated with sexual deviance and social stigma such as HIV/AIDS, the spontaneous improvisation associated with folk media frees participants from society's norms and obligations. As James Ng'ombe concludes, if the common people have been able to create folk art, folk music or folk dances, it makes it imperative to view folk media as an effective strategy for communicating with local communities in development work.[15] In spite of these apparent successes, however, folk media still remain an appendage in most applied-theatre projects. Quite often, it is relegated to the instrumental category of 'folklore', hence commands less serious attention than external artistic conventions.

Participation

Like folk media, participation is another aesthetic category that has also been used and abused for development purposes. As a result, different notions of participation have emerged which can only serve to confuse rather than clarify the concept. As Majid Rahnema elaborates,

> Modern jargon uses stereotyped words [… which] fit arbitrarily together and support the most fanciful constructions. As these words are separate (depending on) context, they are ideal for manipulative purposes. 'Participation' belongs to this category of words.[16]

Several reasons have been put forward for the increased interest in participation by national governments and development institutions since the 1970s.[17] Some of these reasons are:

- bringing greater productivity at low cost;
- being sensitive to the needs and aspirations of the people;
- creating long term sustainability in development;
- readiness to incorporate the local knowledge of the people;

---

[15] Ng'ombe, "The Communication Model and Folk Media in Development."

[16] Majid Rahnema, "Participation," in *The Development Dictionary*, ed. Wolfgang Sachs (London: Zed, 1992): 116.

[17] Rahnema, "Participation"; Nelson & Wright, "Participation and Power"; Chambers, "Paradigm Shifts and the Practice of Participatory Research and Development."

- being a good fund raising device for development agencies;
- allowing more space for the sharing of resources by stakeholders.

However, because of its susceptibility to manipulation, Karl Polanyi argues that participation has been disembedded from its socio-cultural roots and perceived as a 'thing' or 'resource' for keeping the neoliberal global economy alive.[18]

According to Tim Prentki, the global imposition of the neo-liberal economic agenda has resulted in significant aspects of human life being reduced to business transactions.[19] People are defined by who they are, what they own, and how much they have. Those with nothing are excluded not only from economic participation but also from other spheres such as politics, education, science, and technology. In short, human worth has been subordinated to a commercial enterprise. Sheila Preston remarks that it is difficult to achieve genuine participation in such a politicized economic environment because of complex agendas, power relations and competing ideologies.[20] More often than not, the powerful economic forces tend to impose their hegemony on the less powerful. Participation has thus served to reproduce the hegemony of dominant powers. As a result, development workers and applied-theatre practitioners become embroiled in the hegemonic ideology of the neo-liberal value-system rather than transforming it.

However, with the recent shift from a 'top-down' to a 'bottom-up' development approach, participation has begun to shift from 'things' to 'people'. As Robert Chambers points out, "the paradigm of people implies the use of participation (as) an empowering process with a shift of power to those who are local and poor."[21] Its point of departure is characterized by *process* rather than product, *partnership* rather than patronage, and *diversity* instead of uniformity. In the case of applied theatre, this implies that participation has to be *liberating* in order to allow originality of thinking, acting, and feeling in the participants. This view may be compared with John O'Toole's argument

---

[18] In Rahnema, "Participation."

[19] Tim Prentki, "Applied theatre in a global village," in *The Applied Theatre Reader*, ed. Tim Prentki & Sheila Preston (London & New York: Routledge, 2009): 364–65.

[20] Sheila Preston, "Introduction to participation," in *The Applied Theatre Reader*, ed. Tim Prentki & Sheila Preston (London & New York: Routledge, 2009): 127.

[21] Robert Chambers, *Whose Reality Counts? Putting the Last First* (London: IT Publications, 1997).

for integral participation in educational drama.[22] O'Toole identifies three categories of participation: (i) extrinsic participation – where the audience provides feedback during post-performance discussions; (ii) peripheral participation – the audience contributes to the theatrical experience without affecting its structure; and (iii) integral participation – the audience perspective becomes an integral part of the theatrical process. From these categories, O'Toole argues that the most effective way is to structure participation in such a way that it becomes an integral part of the intervention process.

But the contradiction remains that even though there seems to be a shift towards a more empowering brand of popular participation, the neo-liberal paradigm of 'things' remains strong. Perhaps the reason lies in the paradoxes inherent in the term 'participation', which seem to open it up to different interpretations. Even within applied theatre itself, one will be at pains to come up with concrete evidence that indicates that popular participation has succeeded in bringing about local community empowerment. As Majid Rahnema argues, participation cannot be meaningful unless those participating come from a free and unbiased place, yet most societies are based on accepted ideologies that render no one completely free and unbiased.[23] In Sheila Preston's view, any form of participation can either run the risk of reproducing the very hegemony that the project seeks to fight or it may counter such hegemony.[24]

Syncretism

Syncretism has been described as the blending of performance materials and practices from two or more cultural traditions, producing qualitatively new forms.[25] As a dramaturgical strategy, syncretism involves combining local performance idioms with external artistic conventions such as Western theatre to produce hybridized significations. Quite often, syncretism is applied to cultural representations that are aimed at shedding light on the dynamics of a society in transition. As an artistic concept, the paradox of syncretism lies in producing what Christopher Balme has described as "the predicament of

[22] John O'Toole, *Theatre in Education: New objectives for theatre – new techniques in education* (London: Hodder & Stoughton, 1976).

[23] Rahnema, "Participation."

[24] Preston, "Introduction to participation," 128.

[25] David Coplan, *In Township Tonight: South Africa's Black City Music and Theatre* (London: Longman, 1985): vii.

binary cultural encounters,"[26] a condition of unequal interaction between local knowledge-systems and external artistic conventions. As the Japanese theatre practitioner Tadashi Uchino points out, there has been some cross-cultural traffic of theatre practices between Western and Japanese traditions, but this has occurred at the level of appropriation, acculturation, and assimilation rather than dialogue, accommodation, and reciprocity.[27]

Rustom Bharucha has argued against the idea of interculturalism as a corollary of syncretism.[28] He warns that cultural syncretism can become an ethnocentric practice that is not separate from the history of colonialism. More often than not, the specificities of local cultures are submerged by the adoption of an essentialist view of the Other. In the context of an increasingly globalized world where new kinds of identities are being generated, the contradictions of syncretism are no different from those associated with participation. Rather than privileging cultural specificity, reciprocity, and diversity, syncretism has often entailed close identification with the dominant discourse. Through acculturation to neo-liberal ideals of a 'better life' premised on the accumulation of capital, property, and other consumerist products, participants are inclined to be contemptuous of the local in favour of the global. In the words of David George, "reciprocity is as much a political and ethical priority as an aesthetic choice."[29] In other words, one can choose to domesticate rather than accommodate or reciprocate the aesthetic preferences of the Other.

Although the shift towards genuine syncretism in applied-theatre practice has not yet been fully realized, it is important to note that the blending of 'outside-in' (or top-down) and inside-out' (or bottom-up) intervention strategies in contemporary development discourse is sowing the seeds of what

---

[26] Christopher Balme, *Decolonizing the Stage: Theatrical Syncretism and Postcolonial Drama* (Oxford: Clarendon, 1999): 11.

[27] Tadashi Uchino, "Playing Betwixt and Between: Intercultural Performance in the Age of Globalisation," in *Playing Betwixt and Between: The IDEA Dialogues*, ed. Björn Rasmussen & Anna Lena–Ostern (Bergen: IDEA Publications, 2000.

[28] Rustom Bharucha, *Theatre and the World: Performance and the Politics of Culture* (London: Routledge, 1993).

[29] David George, "Reorientations: The Sound of Two Hands Clapping," in *Dis/ Orientations: Cultural Praxis in Theatre: Asia, Pacific, Australia*, ed. Rachel Fensham & Peter Eckersall (Monash Theatre Papers 1; Clayton, Victoria: Centre for Drama and Theatre Studies, Monash University, 1999): 22.

Bjorn Rasmussen and Anna Lena–Ostern have called "playing between and betwixt sameness and difference."[30] This is an intercultural performance paradigm involving a synthesis of different intervention approaches. Practitioners adapt their artistic strategies to suit local performance idioms. Such localisms are re-imagined, re-vitalized, and revised in the process of sharing with the outside world. Thus, applied-theatre performances such as Amakhosi's *Vikela* and DramAidE's *See You at 7* can be seen as forms of intercultural exchange between 'outsiders' (external facilitators) and 'insiders' (target audience).

For example, Amakhosi Theatre has demonstrated a remarkable shift towards syncretism by taking its Theatre for Community Action (TCA) model to the wider Southern African Development Community (SADC).[31] The peoples of the six SADC countries who were involved in the Integrated Regional Development Program (IRDP) – Zimbabwe, Botswana, South Africa, Swaziland, Lesotho, and Mozambique – share only a Nguni dialectal past which has since been distorted by history. Yet, through Amakhosi's TCA intervention model, in particular through localized renditions of its HIV/AIDS play *Vikela*, the different regional communities managed to relate to each other from the vantage of their own cultural diversity. For each of them, difference has not been less a liability than a source of cultural enrichment, a process of learning about HIV/AIDS through aesthetic hybridity.

Since its inception in 1992, DramAidE has been collaborating with an intercultural network of local and global partners in HIV/AIDS education. Its ultimate goal has been to create peer educators who are involved in promoting effective life-skills and positive-behaviour models.[32] In its Annual Report for 2004 and 2005, DramAidE reports that they have been able to team up with global partners such as the Johns Hopkins University Centre for Communication (USA) in the Health Promoters Project, the United States Agency for International Development (USAID) in the Preventing Mother to Child Transmission Project, and the Norwegian Students Academy International Helpfund (SAIH). This is not to mention other collaborative ventures with

---

[30] *Playing Betwixt and Between: The IDEA Dialogues*, ed. Björn Rasmussen & Anna Lena–Ostern (Bergen: IDEA Publications, 2002).

[31] Kennedy Chinyowa, "Helping Them to Help Themselves: Case Study of an Integrated Popular Theatre Approach," *RiDE: Research in Drama Education* 12.2 (June 2007): 133–47.

[32] Dalrymple, "DramAidE: An evaluation of interactive drama and theatre for HIV/AIDS education in South Africa."

local organizations such as the Human Sciences Research Council (HSRC), the Centre for AIDS Development Research (CADRE) and the African Medical Research Foundation (AMREF). In these local community outreach projects, DramAidE and its affiliate partners have followed the principle of unity in diversity through their respect for cultural specificity as an ethical priority. As Richard Schechner points out, the performance of theatre, dance, music, and ritual, by the very nature of their existence as modes of 'restored behaviour', gives us our best example of the field of human communication.[33] These performance genres provide a platform for sharing ideas across intra- and inter-cultural divides.

As with all forms of exchange, however, syncretism also implies negating and neglecting the glaring imbalances and inequalities in power relations between the local and the global. It tends to mask cultural differences in the name of accommodation rather than mutuality. As postcolonial theorists have argued in relation to hybridity,[34] concepts that emphasize cultural exchange often overlook, if not neglect, specific local differences. Needless to say, globalized discourses continue to hold more sway over local knowledge systems in applied-theatre practice.

Conclusion

If one agrees with Cecily O'Neill's assertion that both process and product are part of the same domain, that is, each cannot be extricated from the other in terms of composition, delivery, and reception,[35] then the negative contradictions that are affecting applied theatre as *process* do not augur well for HIV/AIDS education. They paint a rather disquieting picture of the futility of most of the interventions that are meant to solve the plight of those affected and/or infected by the pandemic. It is perhaps because of these contradictions that other applied-theatre critics have not been able to see encouraging prospects for applied-theatre practice. For instance, Helen Nicholson views

---

[33] *The Future of Ritual: Writings on Culture and Performance*, ed. Richard Schechner (London & New York: Routledge, 1993).

[34] For example, *The Postcolonial Studies Reader*, ed. Bill Ashcroft, Gareth Griffiths & Helen Tiffin (London: Routledge, 1999).

[35] Cecily O'Neill, *Drama Worlds: A Framework for Process Drama* (Portsmouth NH: Heinemann. 1995): xvi.

applied theatre as a gift with its own paradoxes.[36] She explains that because this 'gift' can be seen simultaneously as both a 'present' and a 'poison', it is worth remembering that such a present, even if well-intentioned, may be thought to be poisonous by those who live in a different context, and whose version of a 'good life' differs from that of the gift-givers.

The question is: What can be done? The conflict-theorist Peter Coleman has argued that the best method of dealing with intractable conflicts such as race, gender, class, and ethnicity is to acknowledge and confront them.[37] This essay shows how the poetics of applied theatre remain trapped at the crossroads between the aspirations of local communities and the global expectations of practitioners and donor organizations. For instance, the application of aesthetics associated with folk media, participation, and syncretism in HIV/AIDS interventions has tended to create confusing states of 'bewilderment' among practitioners and their intended beneficiaries.[38] Such uncertainty can be overcome by confronting the source of the contradictions. If, for instance, HIV/AIDS interventions are failing because of the hidden agendas of practitioners and donors, then the two should collaborate and resolve their contradictions for the sake of their target audience.

WORKS CITED

Ahmed, Syed Jamil. "Examining interventionist theatre in a multi-axial world of transience: An essay in refusal," in *Drama as Social Intervention*, ed. Michael Balfour & John W. Somers (Concord, Ontario: Captus University Publications, 2006): 40–55.

Ashcroft, Bill, Gareth Griffiths & Helen Tiffin, ed. *The Postcolonial Studies Reader* (London: Routledge, 1999).

Balfour, Michael. "The politics of intention: looking for a theatre of little changes," *RiDE: Research in Drama Education* 14.3 (August 2009): 347–59.

Balme, Christopher. *Decolonizing the Stage: Theatrical Syncretism and Postcolonial Drama* (Oxford: Clarendon, 1999).

---

[36] Helen Nicholson, *Applied Drama: The Gift of Theatre* (Houndmills: Palgrave Macmillan, 2005): 161–62.

[37] Peter T. Coleman, "Intractable conflict," in *The Handbook of Conflict Resolution: Theory and Practice*, ed. Peter T. Coleman & Morton Deutsch (San Francisco: Jossey–Bass, 2000).

[38] James Thompson, *Applied Theatre: Bewilderment and Beyond* (Oxford: Peter Lang, 2006).

Bharucha, Rustom. *Theatre and the World: Performance and the Politics of Culture* (London: Routledge, 1993).

Byam, Dale. *Community in Motion: Theatre for Development in Africa* (Westport CT: Bergin & Garvey, 1999).

Chambers, Robert, "Paradigm shifts and the practice of participatory research and development," in *Power and Participatory Development: Theory and Practice*, ed. Nici Nelson & Susan Wright (London: Intermediate Technology, 1995): 30–42.

——. *Whose Reality Counts? Putting the Last First* (London: IT Publications, 1997).

Chinyowa, Kennedy. "Helping Them to Help Themselves: Case Study of an Integrated Popular Theatre Approach," *RiDE: Research in Drama Education* 12.2 (June 2007): 133–47.

Coleman, Peter T. "Intractable conflict," in *The Handbook of Conflict Resolution: Theory and Practice*, ed. Peter T. Coleman & Morton Deutsch (San Francisco: Jossey–Bass, 2000): 428–50.

Coplan, David. *In Township Tonight: South Africa's Black City Music and Theatre* (London: Longman, 1985).

Dalrymple, Lynn. *A Drama Approach to AIDS Education: A Report on an AIDS and Lifestyles Education Project Undertaken in a Rural School in Zululand* (Kwa-Dlangezwa: University of Zululand, 1992).

——. "The DramAidE Project," in *Drama, Culture and Empowerment: The IDEA Dialogues*, ed. John O'Toole & Kate Donelan (Brisbane: IDEA Publications, 1996): 33–36.

——. "DramAidE: An evaluation of interactive drama and theatre for HIV/AIDS education in South Africa," in *Drama as Social Intervention*, ed. Michael Balfour & John W. Somers (Concord, Ontario: Captus University Publications, 2006): 195–206.

——, ed. "Is DramAidE Making a Difference? Evaluations of DramAidE, Report for Department of Health," in *Monitoring and Evaluation Handbook* (KwaDlangezwa: University of Zululand, 1995).

——, & Paul Botha. *A Facilitator's Guide to See You at 7* (KwaDlangezwa: Atlas Printers, 2001).

Darder, Antonia, Marta Baltodano & Rodolfo Torres, ed. *Critical Pedagogy Reader* (London & New York: RoutledgeFalmer, 2003).

Escobar, Arturo. *Encountering Development: The Making and Unmaking of the Third World* (Princeton NJ: Princeton UP, 1995).

George, David. "Reorientations: The Sound of Two Hands Clapping," in *Dis/Orientations: Cultural Praxis in Theatre: Asia, Pacific, Australia*, ed. Rachel Fensham & Peter Eckersall (Monash Theatre Papers 1; Clayton, Victoria: Centre for Drama and Theatre Studies, Monash University, 1999): 17–29.

Giroux, Henry. *Border Crossings: Cultural Workers and the Politics of Education* (New York & London: Routledge, 1992).

Kamlongera, Christopher. *Theatre for Development in Africa with Case Studies from Malawi and Zambia* (Bonn: German Foundation for International Development, 1988).

Kidd, Ross, & Martin Byram. "Demystifying Pseudo-Freirian Non-Formal Education: A Case Description and Analysis of Laedza Batanani," *Community Development Journal* 17.2 (1982): 91–105.

Luke, Allan, & Carmen Luke. "A Situated Perspective on Cultural Globalisation," in *Globalisation and Education: Critical Perspectives*, ed. N.C. Burbules & C.A. Torres (London: Routledge, 2000): 275–97.

McLaren, Peter. *Critical Pedagogy and Predatory Culture* (New York & London: Routledge, 1995).

Nelson, Nici, & Susan Wright. "Participation and Power," in *Power and Participatory Development: Theory and Practice*, ed. Nici Nelson & Susan Wright (London: Intermediate Technology, 1995): 1–18.

Ng'ombe, James L. "The Communication Model and Folk Media in Development," in *Sustainable Development Dimensions* (Food and Agricultural Organisation (FAO), 2000), http://www.fao.org/sd/CDdirect/CDan0029.htm (accessed 28 July 2011).

Nicholson, Helen. *Applied Drama: The Gift of Theatre* (Houndmills: Palgrave Macmillan, 2005).

O'Neill, Cecily. *Drama Worlds: A Framework for Process Drama* (Portsmouth NH: Heinemann, 1995).

O'Toole, John. *Theatre in Education: New Objectives for Theatre – New Techniques in Education* (London: Hodder & Stoughton, 1976).

Prentki, Tim. "Applied theatre in a global village," in *The Applied Theatre Reader*, ed. Tim Prentki & Sheila Preston (London & New York: Routledge, 2009): 363–67.

Preston, Sheila. "Introduction to participation," in *The Applied Theatre Reader*, ed. Tim Prentki & Sheila Preston (London & New York: Routledge, 2009): 127–29.

Rahnema, Majid. "Participation," in *The Development Dictionary*, ed. Wolfgang Sachs (London: Zed, 1992): 116–31.

Rasmussen, Björn, & Anna Lena–Ostern, ed. *Playing Betwixt and Between: The IDEA Dialogues* (Bergen: IDEA Publications, 2000).

Schechner, Richard, ed. *The Future of Ritual: Writings on Culture and Performance* London & New York: Routledge, 1993).

Thompson, James. *Applied Theatre: Bewilderment and Beyond* (Oxford: Peter Lang, 2006).

Uchino, Tadashi. "Playing Betwixt and Between: Intercultural Performance in the Age of Globalisation," in *Playing Betwixt and Between: The IDEA Dialogues*, ed. Björn Rasmussen & Anna Lena–Ostern (Bergen: IDEA Publications, 2000).

UNESCO. *The Cultural Dimension of Development: Towards a Practical Approach* (Paris: UNESCO, 1995).

van der Stichele, Philippe. "Folk and traditional media for rural development: a workshop held in Malawi," in *Sustainable Development Dimensions* (Food and Agricultural Organisation (FAO), (2000), http://www.fao.org/sd/CDdirect/CDan0029.htm (accessed 28 July 2011).

⌘

JAMIE LACHMAN

Project Njabulo

Using Storytelling, Drama, and Play Therapy for Psycho-Social Interventions in Communities Affected by HIV/AIDS in Southern Africa – Pathways to Empathetic Locally Sustainable Care

Prologue – A Story of Patience

PATIENCE IS A 24-YEAR-OLD WOMAN living in the community of Sinyanmanthula in southeastern Swaziland – an area plagued by severe drought, economic depression, and an HIV prevalence of over 45% of adults. All her family members had recently passed away from HIV/AIDS, leaving her with no home to live in. At the same time, two very young children aged eight and ten were orphaned and left alone in their home. The community elders of Sinyanmanthula responded to the situation by deciding it would be best for Patience to take care of the children. She needed a place to live; the children needed a caregiver. Soon afterwards, however, the community realized that Patience was not taking good care of the children. They were dirty, malnourished, and wearing ragged clothes. Needless to say, they were not happy. The breakdown in family structures had led to a dysfunctional dependency between Patience and the children. A dependency that was devoid of empathic care, compassion, and love.

Background of Clowns Without Borders South Africa

History

Clowns Without Borders was founded in Barcelona in July 1993 when Tortell "Jauma" Poltrona, a professional Catalan clown, was invited to perform in a refugee camp in Croatia. Upon his return to Spain, Jauma founded Clowns Without Borders as a means to provide psychological relief to children affected by crisis. The idea of clowning without borders quickly spread to France, Sweden, and Belgium as artists performed in the Balkans as well as the Middle East and Latin America. By 2000, there were five different CWB chapters, including the USA and Canada, with over a hundred expeditions launched.

In 2003, the South African-born clown and facilitator Jamie McLaren Lachman met Moshe Cohen, the founder of CWB-USA, at a workshop in New York City. He was instantly captivated with the concept of awakening joy and laughter in the hearts of children back in his home country. A year later, Lachman and three clowns from the USA and Ireland journeyed to Southern Africa for a three-week tour. It was an epic trip working with over fifteen different organizations and performing over twenty times for more than 3,000 children in Gauteng, Mpumalanga, KwaZulu–Natal, Free State, and the Western Cape.

Following this expedition, Lachman created Project Njabulo to focus on children affected by HIV/AIDS in Southern Africa. He expanded CWB Project Njabulo in 2005 and 2006 to almost half a year of activity in the field, including projects in Lesotho and Swaziland. At this point, all of CWB Project Njabulo's funding came from the generosity of individuals in the USA. Over this period, they reached more than 60,000 beneficiaries.

While working on a cultural-exchange project between Swedish and South African arts organizations in Durban, 2007, Lachman met many local artists – both professional and amateur youth. These artists came together with Lachman to initiate Clowns Without Borders South Africa. The first project involved an exploratory expedition in partnership with CWB-USA in the Eastern Cape and KwaZulu–Natal with eight artists and facilitators performing eight shows for over 8,000 children. CWBSA followed this trip with an adaptation of Project Njabulo intervention methods to create the Njabulo HIV/AIDS Residency and Life Dreams Follow-Up Programmes in KwaZulu–Natal with the Woza Moya Project and the Rob Smetherham Bereavement Service for Children. This deepened our ability to provide lasting psychosocial support to children and their guardians beyond the momentary relief of performances and one-day workshops.

In 2008, CWBSA expanded its projects to reach over 40,000 beneficiaries with 100 performances and residencies for almost a thousand children and 120 adults. In partnership with our sister CWB chapter in Sweden, we initiated a year-round local-capacity building project in Swaziland with the Lutheran Development Service. We also continued to send residencies and performances to communities in KwaZulu–Natal, Limpopo, Lesotho, and Swaziland with existing and new partners. In order to expand our own capacity, we also began a professional development programme with local youth artists in Durban that addressed issues of xenophobia in response to the violence in May 2008. It was during this time that we received sponsorship from Europcar (formerly Imperial Car Rental) for ground transportation, thereby expanding our capacity to reach more communities.

2009 saw a continuation of CWBSA's growth; we established a local office in Durban and began three additional local capacity building projects in KwaZulu–Natal and Lesotho. We also doubled our operating budget each year, receiving grants from ArtAction, the National Arts Council, PEPFAR (through Ingwavuma Orphan Care), Yale University, the Canadian International Development Agency (CIDA), and the Ethekwini Municipality. From 2011 onwards, CWBSA has also worked in areas outside of Southern Africa, including the Middle East and Sudan.

Since our inception in 2004, CWBSA has provided interventions for over 140,000 children in performances and for more than 1,500 orphans and vulnerable children and caregivers in workshops.

Programmes

CWBSA has the following programmes in its intervention strategy:

1. Performances for Marginalized Communities Affected by Crisis
2 Njabulo HIV/AIDS Residency Programme – Psychosocial Support for Orphans and Vulnerable Children and their Guardians
3 Community Youth Theatre and Empowerment
4 Social Circus Programmes for Affected Children
5 Local Artist Development
6 Community Capacity Building
7 Raising Awareness
8 Monitoring and Evaluation

Who we are

At this point, it is important to emphasize that the aesthetic of clown performance in Clowns Without Borders is derived from traditions of physical comedy in both Western and African contexts. Unlike the stereotypical birthday clown, the clowns come from a background of physical theatre and circus, with many other artforms such as singing, music, dance, puppetry, rhythm, and physical art being incorporated in the work. Further, owing to the holistic nature of our programmes, Clowns Without Borders does not limit participation in projects to artists only but also includes facilitators. As a result, we think of ourselves as 'facilitating artists' who move seamlessly between the worlds of performance and arts education.

Why Clown Performance/Education?

The art of the clown is an essential aspect in all of our work. Whether in performance or in workshops, facilitating artists embody the spirit of play and humour to connect with audience members and participants on a participatory, democratic, and anti-didactic level. There is an element of acceptance and humility in the clown that permeates our work. The clown exists *for* the audience; there is no fourth wall or division between the performer and the audience – the laughter exists between the performer and the audience. As the clown must read and understand its audience, our facilitators are trained to respond to the immediate needs of the participants and adapt when necessary. Furthermore, the humour that is inherent to clown and play opens doors and opportunities to transformation. There is a powerful potential of laughter for cathartic emotional healing. Clowns have been effective in relieving suffering in clinics, refugee camps, hospitals, and hospices. Likewise, laughter is alive throughout our workshops and performances by connecting to the joy of play. Finally, our artistic and pedagogical aesthetic is grounded in improvisation. In clown art, one must be completely vulnerable and resilient in the present moment in order to *play what is happening* and to *be funny*. It is a world in which anything is possible. When something unexpected arises, it is the task of the clown to find a way to *play* with whatever it is. Likewise, our facilitators help participants to discover the means to respond to difficulty with ease and acceptance in order to take the necessary steps and decisions to recover and move forward. As a result, like the clown at every level, CWBSA's work comes from the heart and is offered freely to the community without demanding anything in return.

Providing Psycho-Social Support (PSS) through Arts Interventions to Children and Guardians Affected by HIV/AIDS

Development of intervention model

CWBSA has developed our PSS intervention model, the Njabulo HIV/AIDS Residency Programme, through an organic evolution of programmatic implementation over the past five years using principles of participatory-action research (Figure 1).

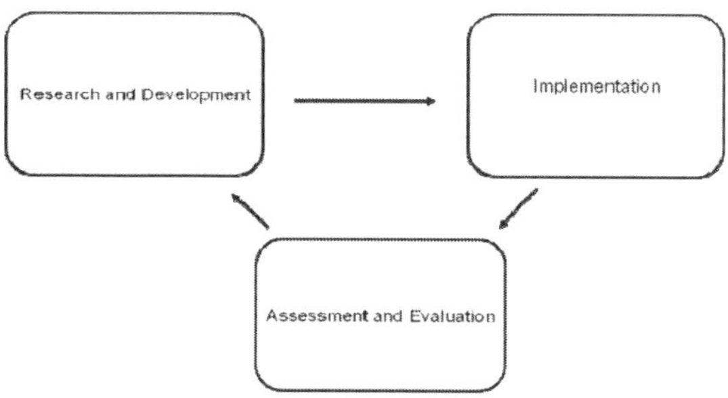

Figure 1: CWBSA participatory action research methodology

This cycle of research–implementation–reflection was essential in formulating an intervention methodology that could respond to the needs of our beneficiaries. By incorporating existing research publications, partner and beneficiary feedback, and internal evaluations, we developed a more accurate picture of the situation for families affected by HIV/AIDS in Southern Africa and how our interventions might have a positive impact. Because CWBSA is primarily an artist-based organization, we relied on a number of studies and consultations with professionals from the fields of psychology and sociology. In particular, a study by the Human Sciences Resource Council published by the Bernard Van Leer Foundation, called *Where the Heart Is*, was extremely influential in the beginning stages of our project development.[1] Likewise, the experience of the Regional Psychosocial Support Initiative was helpful in understanding the psycho-social effects of trauma caused by HIV/AIDS.

---

[1] Linda Richter, Geoff Foster & Lorraine Sherr, *Where the Heart Is: Meeting the Psychosocial Needs of Young Children in the Context of HIV/AIDS* (The Hague: Bernard van Leer Foundation, 2006).

We began by assessing the PSS needs of communities by asking three basic questions:

1. Who were our target beneficiaries?
2. What was the situation and PSS problems facing them?
3. What could we do given our limited resources?

Beneficiaries

Clowns Without Borders South Africa is adamantly against the prevalent dehumanization of humanitarian aid recipients into acronyms. As a result, we resist temptation to refer to orphans and vulnerable children as 'OVCs'. In fact, HIV/AIDS and poverty have affected a wide variety of children – all of whom are vulnerable in Southern African rural society. Many of these children are orphans, living with HIV themselves, living with foster children who are orphans, and caring for sick and dying parents.[2] Likewise, we found that the guardians of the children also are struggling to provide emotional and material support to their children. Many are elderly women, relatives, friends, or neighbours living on the edge of poverty and unable to cope with the extra economic burden of additional children. They are also suffering from losing a loved one from HIV/AIDS and find themselves disconnected from the experience of childcare due to age and grief. As a result, we needed to expand our programme to have a community-wide approach while still focusing on the most vulnerable – children and guardians who are part of our community partners' existing support programmes.

Chronic Psycho-Social Trauma of HIV/AIDS

There are many studies of the psycho-social trauma associated with HIV/AIDS. Our main resource was the work done by the Regional Psychosocial Support Initiative (REPSSI). They found that, in addition to the pre-existing pressure of poverty, there is considerable chronic trauma associated with the HIV/AIDS pandemic. This includes family disintegration, witnessing the death of a loved one, malnutrition and sleep deprivation, inability to pay school fees, and social stigma and discrimination on the part of peers. These sources of trauma combine to have many adverse psycho-social effects on the

---

[2] Richter et al., *Where the Heart Is*, 19.

lives of children, from low self-esteem, chronic depression, and apathy to reduction in coping skills and resilience. Many children withdraw from social interaction and become involved in drug abuse and/or criminal behaviour, resulting in an increased risk of HIV/AIDS infection.[3] Clowns Without Borders began to see this as a cycle of suffering:

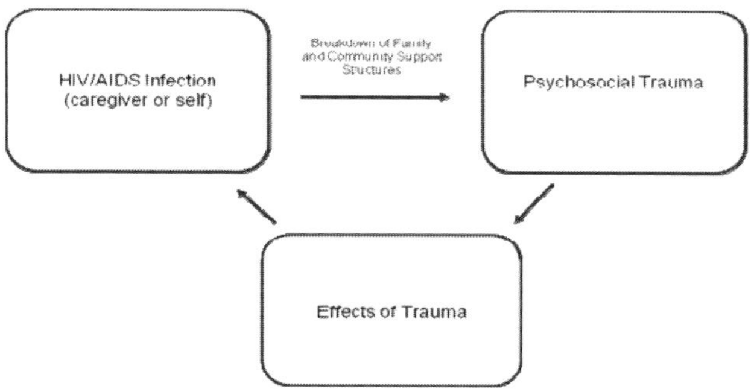

Figure 2: Cycle of Suffering from HIV/AIDS pandemic

Time after time, we needed to remind ourselves that we were not psychotherapists or social workers but artists. Nevertheless, we believed that arts interventions could be utilized to have a positive effect on breaking this cycle of suffering by providing key skills for emotional resilience and recovery to children and guardians. However, before implementing an effective project, we needed to take a closer look at what other organizations were doing as well as our own practices.

Rethinking Our Methods

Clowns Without Borders South Africa's mission is focused on improving the psycho-social well-being of children affected by crisis through play and laughter. Traditionally, our arts interventions consisted of brief visits involving performances at schools and short workshops at drop-in centres or orphanages. However, we soon began to question whether our work was having the impact we desired on the children and, if not, how could we change to better meet the needs of our beneficiaries. In *Where the Heart Is*,

---

[3] Regional Psychosocial Support Initiative, *Psychosocial Care and Support: Mainstreaming Guidelines* (Creative Commons, 2008).

studies showed that interventions that are integrated into existing support structures, in particular on the family level, tend to have a more lasting and beneficial effect on the lives of children. To our dismay, we found that brief interventions that were isolated from other forms of support may actually have an adverse affect by implying that the "community cannot cope on their own [and] erode rather than reinforce resilience that psychosocial programmes aim to strengthen."[4] Furthermore, many humanitarian interventions required a high level of expertise and used foreign intervention methods that failed to resonate in the local cultural context. This resulted in unsustainable practices fuelled by misguided good intentions on the part of many organizations. In fact, on closer inspection, we were forced to admit that Clowns Without Borders was indeed one of these organizations. If we were going to continue working in communities affected by HIV/AIDS in Southern Africa, we needed to have a dramatic shift in our implementation methodology.

Dramatic Shift in Intervention Methodology

Based on our experience and research, in 2008, Clowns Without Borders South Africa made a strategic decision to design a new intervention model using our strengths as artists and facilitators to provide PSS support to children and guardians affected by HIV/AIDS. We decided to implement longer artist residencies instead of performances that focused on strengthening relationships at home. Our new vision was to facilitate empathic interaction between children and guardians that is mutually beneficial while relieving stress and trauma associated with HIV/AIDS. The foundation of our methodology rests on local cultural mediums of storytelling, song, and African drama while integrating innovative techniques such as mindfulness-based stress reduction, play therapy, and symbolic play. We also began to work closely with partner community-based organizations so that our interventions complemented existing support structures such as HIV prevention, food and water security, gender awareness, and paralegal support. Finally, in order to ensure sustainable implementation of our practices, we restructured our methods so that they could be accessible to local-community care-workers and volunteers. As a result, transference of skills to the community level became the central aspect of our intervention strategy in applying the arts to provide lasting PSS to children and guardians affected by HIV/AIDS.

---

[4] Richter et al., *Where the Heart Is*, 33.

Njabulo HIV/AIDS Residency Programme

Performances

Send in the clowns! Over the past eight years, CWBSA has performed for well over 150,000 children and adults in communities affected by crisis. Even though the performances are brief interventions that provide momentary emotional relief, they remain a crucial aspect of our intervention methodology. As an introduction to the community, our performances are a combination of drama, circus, and music that help transform places from grief and emotional suffering to joy and happiness by creating an atmosphere of celebration. Although CWBSA does not focus on direct HIV prevention and education, the performances raise awareness of important issues facing communities relating to the *experience* of being affected by HIV/AIDS. These include discrimination and stigma, poverty, women's empowerment, coping with death, the loss of a loved one, abandonment, and compassion for those who have been affected by the disease. Performances are offered in neutral locations such as public schools and community centres to reduce the stigmatization of children who have been affected by the HIV/AIDS. Thus, the performances create a bridge for the CWBSA facilitating artists to connect immediately with beneficiaries on a broad basis, setting the stage for deeper PSS interventions in residencies.

Residencies

CWBSA's arts education and therapy intervention methodology has been developed specifically for vulnerable children and their guardians affected by HIV/AIDS. Incorporating drama, storytelling, song, circus arts, and mindfulness-based stress reduction, the Njabulo HIV/AIDS Residency Programme (*njabulo* in isiZulu means 'happiness') aims at developing a sense of emotional well-being and resiliency for those who have been directly affected by the pandemic. Participants explore the imagination, play, compassion, gratitude, and lovingkindness through various exercises designed to help them connect to each other at home and thus strengthen the bond between the child and the guardian. Particular attention is given to learning coping mechanisms with stress and grief associated with the loss of a loved one and the burden of poverty. The programme is implemented in two parts: an initial ten-day PSS intervention and a five-day follow-up.

Ten-day initial intervention and five-day follow-up

The initial intervention addresses bereavement and coping skills through a wide variety of applied drama, music, and arts. Working with roughly 35 affected children aged 8–16 and their corresponding guardians, CWBSA facilitating artists lead participants in workshops that explore bereavement issues and parenting skills in a multidiscipline and holistic approach. Our curriculum incorporates traditional cultural mediums of storytelling, song, dance, and African drama with innovative practices of play therapy, symbolic play, circus arts, and mindfulness-based stress reduction. The core focus for the children is to provide a forum to explore bereavement issues and allow them the opportunity to be children again – to play, be creative, and have fun together – in a safe and nurturing environment. The curriculum involves an adaptation of a traditional Southern African story into a dramatic presentation by the children. This story involves themes that are related to the children's lives, including death, dreams, hope, stigma, and community.

At the same time, CWBSA facilitating artists work with the children's primary guardians to develop tools for coping with stress in their lives and also to rediscover a sense of play and creativity through storytelling and games as a way of connecting to their children in a loving relationship. We focus on storytelling, play, and mindfulness-based stress relief in these sessions as well as employing songs, games, and simple movement exercises. The guardians are also given homework each day to begin incorporating storytelling and games into their interaction with the children. They report their successes and difficulties with the homework exercises at the beginning of the following session. The final session focuses on providing tools to continue incorporating storytelling, play, and relaxation beyond the residency. The guardians are instructed in simple techniques of mindfulness-based stress reduction that they can use on a daily basis. They are also invited to the culminating activity of the children's workshop.

Culminating activities

At the end of each residency, the children and guardians come together in a culminating activity, or Family Day, that celebrates the completion of the programme. This event involves all participants in games, traditional dance and song, and other exercises. It is important to provide an opportunity for the children and guardians to play together as well as to share their stories. During the ten-day residency, the children perform an adaptation of a traditional Southern African story that deals with bereavement issues. In the five-day workshop, this performance is transformed into short plays depicting how the children will achieve their life dreams. The guardians also share stories they have created during the residency.

Transference to the Community Level

In order to ensure the sustainability of CWBSA's arts intervention practices beyond the limited scope of our organization, we have begun to implement capacity-building programmes with local community partners in KwaZulu–Natal, Swaziland, and Lesotho. CWBSA has two transference models, the implementation of which depends on the amount of funding and organizational capacity of our partner (Figures 3 and 4). These models involve intense experiential learning for staff members, community care-workers, and volunteers, as well as workshops prior to and following interventions. Both models include an assessment and evaluation of our partner's capacity followed by supplemental training to augment skills. Recognizing the diversity of each area and community organization, these models are by no means rigid but are adaptable to the given circumstances in the field. Nevertheless, the ultimate objective of CWBSA's capacity-building programme is for our community partners to be able to conduct ongoing PSS support groups for children and guardians that meet at least once a month. If necessary, CWBSA continues to provide support and training of community workers to maintain the necessary skills to expand and sustain these support groups.

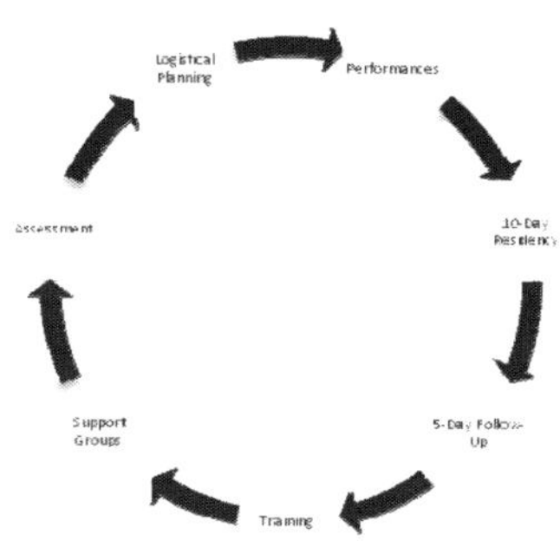

Figure 3: Intervention Model 1: Basic Transference to Community Level

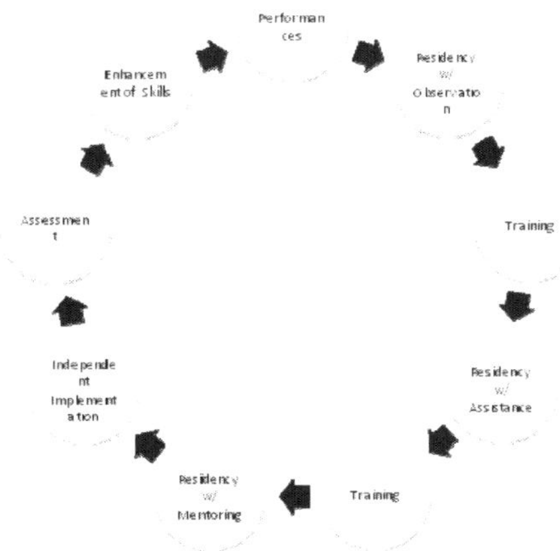

Figure 4: Intervention Model 2: Complete Transference of Skills to Community Level

As mentioned earlier, CWBSA currently has four capacity building projects: two in KwaZulu–Natal with Woza Moya Project and Ingwavuma Orphan Care; one in Lesotho with the Malealea Development Trust; and one in Swaziland with the Lutheran Development Service. After completing full transference of skills to LDS in Swaziland, CWBSA handed over Njabulo Residency implementation to our partners, with UNICEF Swaziland providing additional support to strengthen the sustainability of support groups.

Monitoring and Evaluation

As an integral part of the process of developing intervention practices, CWBSA constantly evaluates and assesses the impact of our activities. Beneficiaries, trainees, partners, and facilitating artists participate in focus groups reflections, individual interviews, baseline surveys, and evaluations following each residency and capacity building project. Furthermore, our community partners conduct follow-up exercises with children and guardians on an ongoing basis in order to assess the impact of our endeavours on their already existing support services. CWBSA has also begun to implement a comprehensive evaluation strategy through baseline surveys of our beneficiaries' psycho-social well-being. We are presently looking for partners from the academic world to help in analysing and publishing our findings, as such dissemination is crucial to our understanding of how we can continue to improve the emotional well-being of children and their caregivers in Southern Africa.

Conclusion – Challenges and a Testimony of Patience

In conclusion, CWBSA's programmes continue to evolve as we learn more about the nature of how arts-based intervention practices can be a powerful tool in providing psycho-social support to children and guardians affected by crisis. We face considerable challenges in balancing innovation with standardization, staff turnover, and funding. Furthermore, although the response to our work on the part communities and partners has been overwhelmingly positive, we have yet to implement a comprehensive PSS evaluation on our methodology. This is a crucial step in analysing and adjusting the curriculum to best serve the communities. However, one can become distracted by incessant reports, evaluations, baselines, and project models, losing sight of the children and guardians. At the end of the day, the simplicity of loving interaction cannot be underestimated. This was especially poignant in the aforementioned story of Patience.

In August 2008, when Clowns Without Borders came to Sinyamathula in collaboration with the Lutheran Development Service, Patience reluctantly joined the Njabulo Residency Program for caregivers and their children. Although she was very shy and rarely talked openly, she attended every session and participated in all the activities with the other caregivers.

During the culminating activity, when the adults were invited to come watch the children act out their story, Patience arrived with her children. We noticed that the children were clean and were holding Patience's hands. In the reflection with the guardians on our last day, Patience began to share her experience openly:

> Being part of this group changed the way I think about the orphans in my care. I used to think of just packing my stuff and leave these children alone. I realized that when doing the awareness activities and body relaxations, I feel better.
>
> I now want to be with my children, to share stories and be close to them and care for them. Before I came to this group I always felt alone in caring for these children. Being here made me realize that I am not alone. There are others who are in the same situation and we can support each other.
>
> Even my children have changed. I can see an easy connection between them and me. Beforehand, they would not come to me when I came home. But now they come freely to me. They share things that they did at school and in the programme. I want to be there for my children. We love each other.

Testimonies such as Patience's speak volumes about the positive impact of our work in connecting children and caregivers in nurturing relationships, and underscores the need for more interventions in the field. Guardians rediscover the benefits of empathic care in their families. And children are once again allowed to be children – to play, to laugh, and to be loved. This is the work and play of Clowns Without Borders South Africa.

Works Cited

Regional Psychosocial Support Initiative. *Psychosocial Care and Support: Mainstreaming Guidelines* (Creative Commons, 2008).

Richter, Linda, Geoff Foster & Lorraine Sherr. *Where the Heart Is: Meeting the Psychosocial Needs of Young Children in the Context of HIV/AIDS* (The Hague: Bernard van Leer Foundation, 2006).

⌘

Innovative Case Studies

MYER TAUB

Dramatic Beading

Background

IN JULY 2009, I WAS AWARDED A DOCTORAL DEGREE in drama for my dissertation entitled "Lessons from an aftermath: recovery of the self through trans-disciplinary applied drama practice." This research applied a combination of elements extracted from across disciplines into a dialogic method of applying drama practice to various non-theatrical sites so as to induce performance research projects, as well as case studies, in order to examine the notion of recovery in the realm of the aftermath: specifically, at first, the September 11 attacks in New York and then, comparatively, the aftermath of apartheid and the aftermath of the advent of HIV/AIDS. The methodology that governed my research projects, occurring first at a high school in Cape Town and then at an HIV/AIDS wellness clinic, also in Cape Town, was framed by a case-study model[1] that I modified to incorporate three stages of research: i) experimental, ii) descriptive, and iii) explanatory. All three stages were re-adjusted according to a heuristic principle[2] that suggests that the discovery of knowledge might occur from within the realm of the unknown. This was an experiential research process which did not separate the subjective self from the researcher's pursuit of collaborative–reciprocal knowledge and reflexive recovery. The actual activation of the research pro

[1] Robert Yin, *Case Study Research: Design and* Methods, vol. 5 (Thousand Oaks CA: Sage, 2003), and *Applications of Case Study* Research, vol. 34 (Thousand Oaks CA: Sage, 2003).

[2] Clark Moustakas, *Heuristic Research: Design, Methodology and Applications* (Thousand Oaks CA & London: Sage, 1990), and *Phenomenological Research Methods* (Thousand Oaks CA & London: Sage, 1994).

jects meant developing a particular kind of template that utilized recovery both as a paradox and as a symbol for self-repair and self-revelation. The template functions by creating projects that integrate the use of interactive narrative combining elements from across the creative-art disciplines to stimulate performing recovery. In November 2009, thanks to subsequent funding from various sources including the National Arts Council of South Africa, I returned to the wellness clinic in Cape Town to continue developing a project called 'Christine's Room'. This project was set up to continue a previous exploratory adaptation of Henrik Ibsen's play *A Doll's House* by integrating site-specific performance, cartography, and video. One of the aims of the project was to have a workshop open to the public on World AIDS Day 2009 in Cape Town.

Revision

First, a digital sequence was reproduced from video documentation made during the first phase of the drama workshop that I facilitated at the Monkeybiz wellness clinic, Cape Town, in November 2005. The image below is a frame of myself and a group of participants in the drama workshop, who are also members of the wellness clinic and beading collective, watching a segment of video from the previous session – so as to watch ourselves doing drama on video and then to extract recognizable dramatic forms. These forms were then practised and reproduced into making live dramatic narratives. There is a voice-over of my voice, re-made during the editing process and re-applied to this particular video segment.

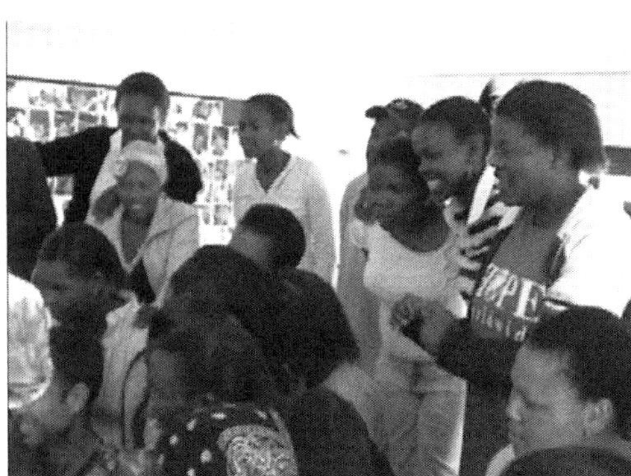

Figure 1: Watching video at the Monkeybiz wellness clinic, Cape Town

This is my voiceover:

> What you do every week or everyday here is that you take beads and put them together, all right, to make something else. To make something bigger, to make a story, those beads are fragments, they are bits and pieces of something and when you put them together you make something else, that's what we each did–each of those things was a bead and we put them all together and made a story and put them in a bag… (11 November 2005)

William Kentridge, in "The mouth of the crocodile," the essay introducing his play text *Ubu and the Truth Commission*, speaks of "a faith in the practical epistemology in the theatre – trusting and using the edifices and techniques of theatre to generate meaning."[3] Kentridge highlights the rehearsal process as an example of practical epistemology in theatre: of how, in rehearsal, the dramatic moment is made – much as meaning might be discovered through a repetitive-replicatory-distillation process. Kentridge's belief that knowledge made through practice and located in something like the revision process is useful at this stage of the present essay, where I return – not only to describe, but also to revise and reflect on – to my previous doctoral research case studies, that occurred specifically at the wellness clinic, but also to demonstrate how returning to make and extract meaning from previous practice informs research and generates and advances future practice. By returning to previous case studies, as a process of revision, I hope to elicit an understanding of how to make meaning for future projects. In particular, this involves the project called 'Christine's Room', the description and explanation of which shall feature in, as well as tentatively shaping, this essay's narrative.

Further, this essay's narrative is an embodiment of assumed reflexivity. By this I mean the ways in which reflexivity occurs through critical re-assessment of and reflection on previous practice, and how this advances practice and explores the assumption that the process itself will progress by turning back. In other words, to adopt the perspective of the anthropologists Barbara Myerhoff and Jay Ruby: "to contemplate ourselves just as we may be beginning to realize that we have no clear idea of what we are doing."[4] This

---

[3] William Kentridge, "The mouth of the crocodile," in *Ubu and the Truth Commission*, ed. Jane Taylor (Cape Town: U of Cape Town P, 1998): 12.

[4] Barbara Myerhoff & Jay Ruby, "A Crack in a Mirror: Reflexive Perspectives in Anthropology," in *Remembered Lives: The Work of Ritual, Storytelling and Growing Older*, ed. Myerhoff & Marc Kaminsky (Ann Arbor: U of Michigan P, 1992): 307.

description suggests something of my own position, of being unclear about what lies ahead in my planning for 'Christine's Room' except that the answers may reside in turning back in order to reflect on and critically assess previous projects. By exposing the integuments of the earlier process, I am retracing steps that, in Jacques Derrida's terms, are like "advancing backwards."[5] So here I am – advancing backwards in a resolve to look for any clues embedded in previous practice and motivated by how returning to this particular project will inspire the process that, in the words of the research activist Donald Schön, becomes a "repetitive or experimental activity – from which occurs a repertoire of expectations, images and techniques,"[6] subsequently merging the process with a research method that encourages practice-led research to be inventive as much as it implies a revision-like method of practice.

In this essay, simultaneously re-searching and presenting previous practice over five years is like presenting a series of experiential repertoires as vignettes or beads that, when strung together, describe the challenges of working in the field of applied drama with a group of Xhosa-speaking craft beaders who are also HIV-positive. It also attempts to explain the process not only of making drama projects from within the wellness clinic but also to bring out the emergence of self-awareness in my capacity as a researcher working in the face of the demands made by disease and politics in postcolonial South Africa.

Self-awareness as part of the subjective paradigm in research suggests using operatives like the self and reflexivity (hence self-reflexivity) as a strategic device to perforate the enclosure, at the same time exemplifying the role of reflexivity as a proactive mechanism in examining practice and generating research.[7] The reflexive exercise might penetrate the representational form –

[5] Jacques Derrida, "The Time Before The First," in *The Derrida Reader: Writing Performances*, ed. Julian Wolfeys (Lincoln: U of Nebraska P, 1988): 130.

[6] Donald Schön, *The Reflective Practitioner: How Professionals Think in Action* (London: Temple Smith, 1983): 60.

[7] Reflection is meditative thinking aboutwhat has occurred before, whereas reflexivity is a corresponding action of reflection – it is both a critical and an ambiguous trajectory, considering its own implications and the presence of subjectivity. Douglas Macbeth's definition of reflexivity – " a deconstructive exercise for locating the intersections of an author, other, text, and world, and for penetrating the representational exercise itself" ("On 'reflexivity" in qualitative research: Two readings and a third," *Qualitative Inquiry* 7.1 [2001]: 35 – is useful for exemplifying reflexivity as a pro-

meaning: also the enclosure, also definition, also the boundary, also an academic kind of narcissism – all of which I would also like to align with Homi Bhabha's description:

> a horizontal mode of thinking that resists integrating a dialectic of possibilities, of different conjectures, the doublings in narratives and complexities in reasoning that exist in a post-colonial landscape.[8]

Thus, when the perforation of the enclosure occurs, there is an endless possibility of meaning. As Bhabha implies, there is "no single explanation sending one back immediately to a single origin is adequate – there are no simple discrete formations or social processes."[9]

The perforation of the enclosure becomes a metaphoric device in and of itself when engaging with HIV/AIDS. Rather than cementing the virus, or resisting its integration, there is reciprocation and meeting – head-on with it, not as an equal but in a rhizomatic way that instead might challenge the virus.

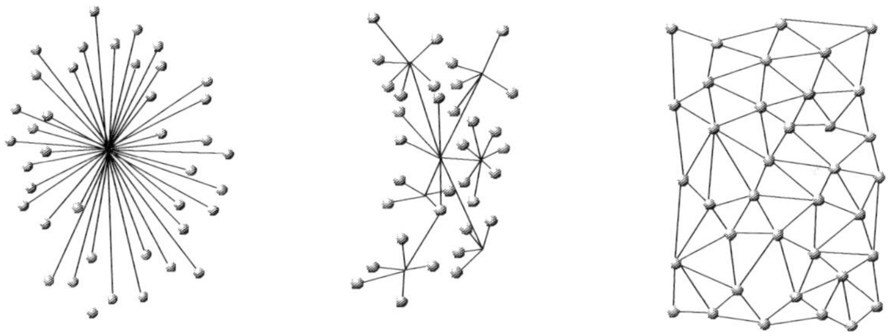

Figure 2: rhizome models[10]

---

active mechanism in examining practice and generating research. Similarly, reflexivity occurs when mirrors double, creating a *mis-en-abyme*: "the endless regress of possibilities," thus advancing the research (Myerhoff & Ruby, "A Crack in a Mirror," 309).

[8] Homi Bhabha, *The Location of Culture* (London: Routledge, 1994): 141.

[9] Bhabha, The Location of Culture, 293.

[10] These models have been adapted from Paul Baran's computer-network diagrams. Baran pointed out that distributed networks are less vulnerable to attack than centralized network structures. His network diagrams are also known in cyber-terminology as "network topologies" – see Paul Green, "Paul Baran and the Origins of the Internet," http://www.rand.org/about/history/baran.html (accessed 22 May 2010), and Martin Dodge, "An Atlas of Cyberspaces," in *Cyber Geography Research* (2007), http://www .personalpagesmanchester.ac.uk (accessed 2008).

Drama is a form that is comparable to the multidimensional form of the rhizome. I originally derived this idea from Gilles Deleuze and Félix Guattari's terminology[11] because theirs resembles drama's multimedial nature. There is a synthesis here between the multi-connections located in a rhizome and the multiple created interactions made from the dynamics of drama. Both drama and the rhizome are heterogeneous; neither "necessarily linguistic."[12] Both evoke multiplicity, both can instigate further evolution and generate different kinds of reception; both can be reproduced and contextualized in alternative types of multi-text such as cartography, performance, and video.

Beading

This essay is called "Dramatic Beading" because it attempts to correlate an application between beading and applied drama practice in the context of the particular HIV/AIDS wellness clinic in Cape Town, as much as it aims to embody a series of experiential repertoires presented as if on a string of beads. To assist in this assemblage is a chronological framework beginning at the end of 2005. In November 2005, I was approached by the Monkeybiz Beading Collective to facilitate an hourly bi-weekly drama workshop for the members of their wellness clinic, which is located in Bo-Kaap, Cape Town and situated above the Monkeybiz Factory Shop. On the surface, the clinic operates like an informal network, but in reality there is a tacit efficiency that provides skills-training and HIV/AIDS support for low-income HIV-positive women. The clinic began in 2003 and caters for approximately seventy women who supply the collective with beading work. Their first language is Xhosa, they are aged between twenty and forty years, and the majority reside in Khayalitsha Township. The clinic offers them beadwork training, a light meal, and basic nutrition instruction in a safe and confidential environment. All who attend the clinic supply the non-profit factory shop with their labour, the fruits of which operate the clinic. There is thus an ethos of assertiveness that recalls Michel Foucault's view:

---

[11] Gilles Deleuze & Félix Guattari, *A Thousand Plateaus: Capitalism and Schizophrenia*, tr. Brian Massumi (*Capitalisme et schizophrénie* 2: *Mille plateaux*, 1980; Minneapolis: U of Minnesota P, 1986).

[12] Victor Taylor & Charles Winquist, *Encyclopedia of Post Modernism* (New York: Routledge, 2001): 343–46.

> in self-financing of the poor themselves [...] indicating a practical objective at best to tackle poverty useful by fixing it to the apparatus of production, at worst to lighten as much the burden it imposes on the rest of society.[13]

What occurs from the overall perspective of the clinic points to relationships of interdependence between the mechanism of the individual and the politics of the collective in order to sustain health. It exists in the interrelationship between the informal structures of the clinic and the formal expectations of commerce. This is evident in the practice of beading. Here the individual might initiate beadwork alone but relies on the collective for the nurturing of the maker of the object in question.[14] Nurturing by the collective includes providing advice, positive critique, and impetus to the individual beader. The collective making their own beadwork in the experience of a communal space such as the clinic accommodate the exchanges between individual and collective.

What links the politics of health care and the cultural politics of beading to the challenges of working in the context of HIV/AIDS in the field of applied drama is finding a way to transcend language barriers. These crises and strategies of mediation determine a redirection of the challenges ahead. Presently, I am offering no solution. Although I suspect that what lies ahead in the reformation of 'Christine's Room' as a project could be a way to negotiate some of the challenges I have already experienced in this field.

Helen Nicholson raises the challenge of dramatic literacy and differentiated knowledge in applied drama.[15] She argues for locating a process of exchange based on differentiated knowledge; locating not only relational exchanges but in the locale of Paolo Freire's word-action; this would then recognize Wittgenstein's maxim (the limits of my language are the limits of my world), and

---

[13] Michel Foucault, "The Politics of Health in the Eighteenth Century" (1976), in *The Foucault Reader*, ed. Paul Rabinow (Harmondsworth: Penguin, 1984): 276.

[14] Beading is a significant historical amalgamation of indigenous African traditional craft and commercial European artifact. Fragments from different cultural codes transcend barriers of *langue* and ethnicity when assembled along new lines. Beading has become an important source of income for the indigent women at the wellness clinic; their beading also sustains the running costs of the clinic, and beading is a form of self-expression, translating traditional craft and transcending language and cultural barriers.

[15] Helen Nicholson, *Applied Drama: The Gift of Theatre* (New York: Palgrave Macmillan, 2005): 51.

understanding how drama practice is a form of literacy "where you can feel through the body, aurally, visually and kinaesthetically."[16] Accommodating the relational exchanges of differentiated vocabulary made in action demonstrates the challenges ahead. Such alternate forms of literacy can occur instantaneously through play, where the body reads, responds, and is read instinctively through a set of unconscious directives operating from within group practice.

Play

From my journal entry dated 25 November 2005:

> Practising the small fragments of action and assembling them into a whole as a short play/skit have become important. We begin today with a warm up, massaging each other's bodies in a circle, rubbing each other's bodies in awkward places so participants laugh and jump at being uncomfortable. We play broken telephone and then rehearse as practicing repetition of the fragment of actions. We don't even have time to watch the video documentation from last week instead we practice what we can remember again and again as a pattern forming a performance. We develop the idea of testimony at the end of the scene where everyone drops the large suitcase they have been carrying on their shoulders or backs and each participant, one after another, enters into the circle and discloses something about themselves. Every participant without any urging from myself chooses to say they are HIV-positive.

In disclosing a verbal artefact as important as one's HIV status, there are enormous resonances in the spheres of ethics, stigma, performance, narration, and testimony. I must make it clear that this action of disclosure came from the participants. All through this first stage of the project, I did not directly confront the collective status of the group. The impetus had been around assembling fragments of action, stories, and sounds inspired by recalling an experience of a broken necklace. The position of the group as participants was now altered by their own need to unpack this important fragment of information; they had initiated agency for themselves of what was important to tell. The disclosure seemed to be an imagined removal of the condition from the body through utterance by purging the body of the fragment, sending it back

[16] Nicholson, *Applied Drama: The Gift of Theatre*, 51–56.

into the ruin – and the need to authenticate the condition through the experience of individual disclosure in the repository of the collective. It is interesting to compare the role of secrets in the process: originally, in the game of broken telephone, the secrets were whispered and conjured up a performativity of dialogic intimacy from one person to another; now, the imagined secrets were openly disclosed and initiated intimacy from one person to everyone. Here, collective solidarity is reinforced through disclosure and supported the occurrence of the disclosure.

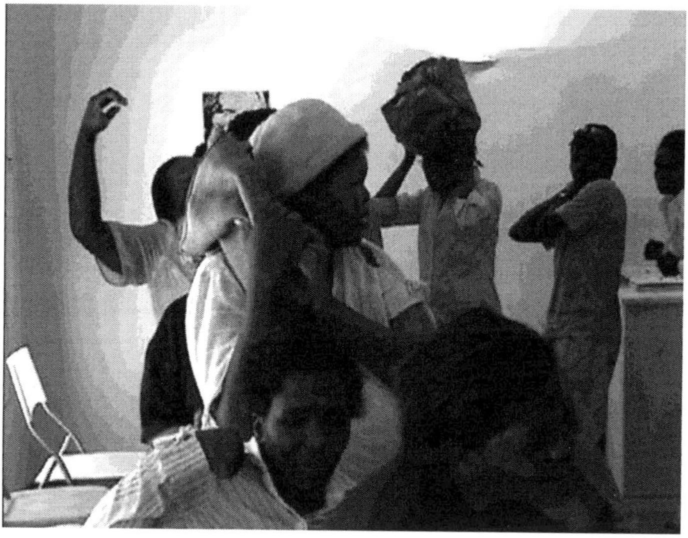

Figure 3: Playing with bags and beads

Early Digital Crisis

I became aware that the documentation on DVD added a different dimension to the process, although, at the same time, I became somewhat suspicious of the message it had begun to generate. On the DVD, the testimony becomes the central focus of this particular meeting. In the experience, the action of performance activated testimony, and not the other way round. This meant that testimony was secondary to performance. In the early stages of this project, I realized how watching the recorded work helped participants to reproduce narratives of action that occurred previously. Participants were at ease in re-creating narratives quickly from this process. Significantly, it seemed that watching one's own action from a distance composed in another medium and thereafter extracting from this in order to reproduce an alternative narrative might ease the stigma of the virus. Producing narrative through digital reproduction engineered a process of dismantling stigma or the debilitating effect of stigma; participants were willing to expose their status publicly. What was significant was how the mechanism of digital reproduction of performance and testimony in performance involved a synergy of dual processes of assembling and dismantling. However, the group began to rely on the digital video as a process of reflection and reproduction, and this process became costly. At the same time, the participants were reluctant to write anything down, even expressing resistance to this. I suspect that this was due to their being self-conscious about their literary proficiency. Instead, they were happy to be filmed during the process, but sometimes the digital work lacked a sufficient sense of engagement of a collaborative process of producing data and exchange of group narratives. I also become aware that through the first stage of this process some of the participants were eager to perform for the camera and less eager to perform for each other as a collective without it. This also occurred the other way round, where some of the participants became more self-conscious once the camera was in the room.

My dilemma with digital video as a medium was not that it could inform pedagogic reproduction, or accommodate a sense of safety, or contribute to valuable archive of documentation; instead, the medium was, in Tri Minh-ha's term, "elastic."[17] This meant working with a medium that was capricious and compressible, flexible and versatile and often unethical; it displaced boundaries but at the same time created new ones. This digital crisis was one of several that occurred in my research and practice at the wellness clinic.

To sum up these crises, I refer to Michelle Fine's "anxieties of dis-integrity"[18] as states of anxiety projected by the researcher onto the subject of research itself. This occurs because of the unconscious anxiety instilled by the researcher's own anxieties about the subject's apparent condition. The point of this crisis in my research was that I unconsciously created and projected my own anxieties and fear of HIV/AIDS onto the women whose bodies and predicament were an example of my anxieties, which were in danger of

[17] Trinh T. Minh-ha, *The Digital Film Event* (London Routledge, 2005): 56.

[18] Michelle Fine, "Working the Hyphens: Reinventing Self and Other in Qualitative Research," in *The Landscape of Qualitative Research: Theories and Issues*, ed. Norman K. Denizen & Yvonna S. Lincoln (Thousand Oaks CA: Sage, 1998): 147.

becoming reinforced. This predicament presented and exacerbated yet another crisis. The attempt to embrace the 'Other' within myself and to acknowledge that I, as a white, Jewish, gay, (HIV-negative), prosperous male, with a specific vocabulary, also wanted to attempt to heal and repel what was the 'Other' (of gender–disease–race) located in the subject – black, Xhosa, Christian, (HIV-positive), indigent, female, and therefore possibly 'dangerous'. Fine does not offer tangible solutions to this crisis except perhaps to "'come clean' about the contradictory stances, politics, perspectives and histories we import to our work."[19]

Allegory and *A Doll's House*: Towards Christine's Room

To sublimate this crisis, I began to do two things: to search for a kind of allegory or metaphor derived from the work that would intervene, position, understand, and construct conversations with moments of crises that fragment the personal; and to search for an alternate form of reproductive method that could replace the digital recording of activities.

In mid-April 2006, in order to extend the idea of allegorical strategy, I decided to extract a particular fragment of text from *A Doll's House*. In the text there is a scene early on in the play when Christine visits her old childhood friend, Nora. In the scene, Ibsen explores issues of illness, secrecy, and stigmatization. At first Nora does not recognize her old friend, because Christine has changed physically through age and possibly illness. Ibsen created a play filled with marginal identities that strive for coexistence and in doing so challenge boundaries of gender and social identities. Boundaries that were once immutable became ambiguous; what appears fixed is now open to adaptation and is thus allegorical. The potential ambiguity encouraged me to introduce the text at the wellness clinic. I had also hoped that doing so would enable the application of a rhizomatic process that might provide a means to explore allegorical extensions as a multiple activity within practice. The outcome was the creation of a physical place and the genesis of a project called 'Christine's Room' – a new context for an original drama. The place that was created was a space between spaces, an interstice that was safe. It told the story of Christine, Nora's friend, left behind and marginalized, a struggling and unfortunate but determined widow, and she lived in an intimate space that represented something of everyone's room. It also had Nora leaving Torvald

[19] Fine, "Working the Hyphens," 148.

and Norway and travelling almost two hundred years to reach Christine's room, now located in the Makhaza settlement of Khayalitsha in Cape Town. In order to reach this room, Nora used a map.

Mapping and the use of the map as a means of navigation in the project meant applying the making of maps: encoding thought and image onto a flattened document with a pen represented a generative–reflective process in the workshops as a whole. Cartography became a process of work in itself and created an avenue of reflection that challenged and replaced digital documentation. It was thus a proposal for 'poor' research that embraced a low-tech, low-maintenance form of documentation and reproduction. This was also 'creative practice' that promoted maps as an alternate text, a form of expression beyond linguistic, cultural, and enclosed boundaries. Maps became a way to chart participants' responses to activities in which they were engaged. This led to the development of new language tools: not only as "a symbol system for mapping the world as it is but as a performative means for co-coordinating activities"[20] to assist in understanding each other.

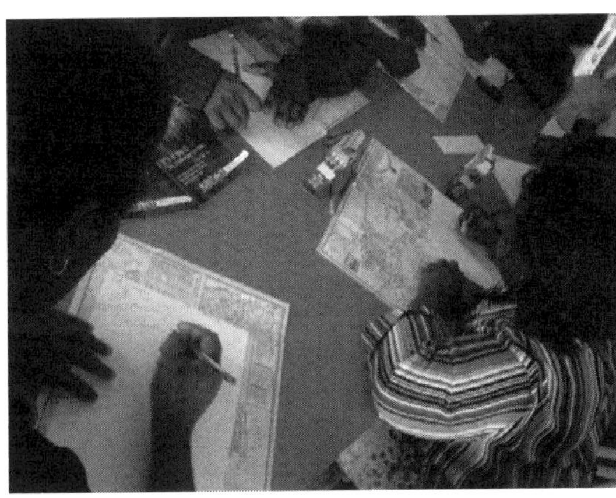

Figure 4: Exploring maps as mapping

[20] Frederick Steier, *Research and Reflexivity* (Thousand Oaks CA & London: Sage, 1991): 51.

Mandisa's Map

Mandisa is one clinic member who was prolific in making maps in the drama workshops. When I asked Mandisa in a group discussion why she was drawing maps, she replied:

> They are maps because it was what we have done so now we have to write it down. The routes we have taken, the things we have done so that's why we call them maps. It is the things we have seen.[21]

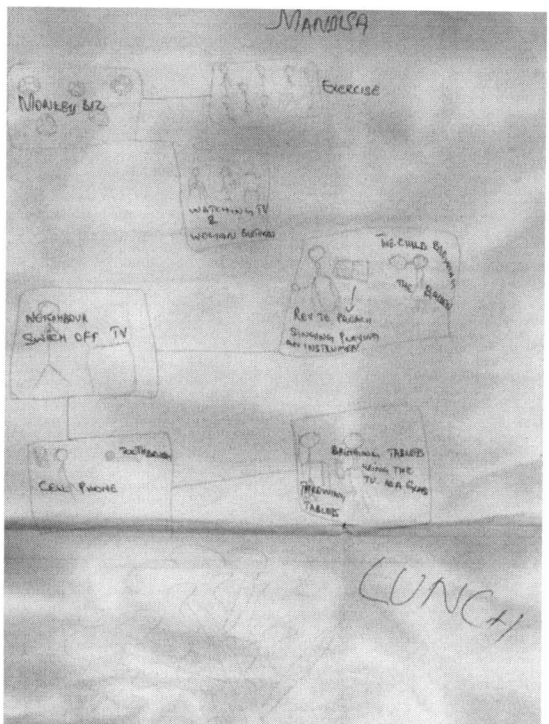

Figure 5: Mandisa's fourth map

Mandisa seems to grasp both method and form, indicated by her use of words made explicit by "routes" and "the things we have done" and "seen." This is an indication of an active advancement in understanding and of agency in regard to this method of mapping. Significantly, the fourth map she made (above) consolidates elements from her previous maps. It is reflective, conclu

---

[21] Excerpt from interview.

sive, and takes on the diagrammatic conventions of maps influenced from the previous day's activities. It summarizes play-making as dramatic narrative, with each unit enlarged with detail: pictures, objects, and inscription. It also has two inscriptions which, although they are not clear on the map as reproduced, are still important to point out. One indicates her earlier referencing of regeneration: "that is growing into a tree and this is something beautiful" and another says: "we are videorized," suggesting awareness and acceptance of other forms of recording methods. I am also aware of how the term suggests not only video but could also allude to invasion perpetrated by an outside force such as a virus. The mapping processes were intriguing and fruitful, and validated my assumptions about alternative modes of communication. Cartography was indispensable and became a predominant mode and medium in every subsequent project.

Re-Mapping Video

Subsequently, since 2006 and then on to the end of my doctoral research in 2008, I used maps as an alternative medium to digital reproduction. But I did not forgo digital documentation completely, relying on it to record outcomes from the mapping process and to maintain the accumulative archive from the practice. Now, as I return to the project, with significant funding, I can also return to video as a complementary, interdependent medium in relation to mapping. How I visualize 'Christine's Room', or the re-creation of *Christine's Room*, is the making of an interactive, travelling space that is assembled in performance by the performers themselves and stores the accumulation of digital documentation as well as digital expression. How I got this point is mapped out in the drama workshops that began again on 23 November at the Monkeybiz wellness clinic.

Thus far, maps have been the documented experience of the research and have generated its subsequent practice. Maps have also consolidated practice as research. But the process has not ended with maps but has been extended by mapping and remapping. Hence, the process that accommodates the already multiple and complex process of practice-led research in a complex terrain accommodates and connects with video. For although video and cartography suggest flat one- and two-dimensional documents, they are also able to represent spatial regions and embody authentic generative-reflective and freshly rehearsed processes. Thus, there is an intersection here, with interplay between these two forms that is fluid and elastic, forming part of a larger process of knowing, memory, and meaning-making, of experience as knowledge, with the enclosure perforated along the way. They are like penetrative rhizomes, much as Deleuze and Guattari describe their rhizomes with their "multiple interpretations and readings, providing more tools, more language and more assemblages to help us think in ways that maps do."[22] I thus continue to plan with and revise ideas generated from previous research and practice in order to remake 'Christine's Room', which is presently to form partly a video archive, partly a large performative mapping of what has occurred before investing the original material in something more sustainable. The aim of the project would be to reveal the indomitable spirit of humanity, with regard both to survival more immediately and, more broadly, to life itself. I continue to visit and teach workshops at the wellness clinic and still face frustration and crises there, but I have realized that I go there because the women teach me things about myself. They constantly inform us of ways in which drama and beading can interrelate and how play can make meaning. Drama and beading are both produced from the body, both engage with a fragment that is assembled, and, in this case, both meet in an aftermath of the advent of HIV/ AIDS. Here, too, drama joins Foucault's imperatives located in the interdependence of individual and collective in the larger framework of politics and health. By placing the wellness clinic in a specific context of public health, I could not ignore the operation of the individual researcher and practitioner, because it is the actions of the collective as much as the merging voices of individuals that reflect the shape of my research process at the clinic, its outcomes, and the nature of future projects. In the above, I have endeavoured to consistently link the interdependency of individual and collective in public health to the cultural politics of beading. I do realize that I have somewhat complicated this link by involving my own practice-led research aims of concurrency. My research, as much as my practice in its overall context, values the multiplicity of theories and the interdisciplinary nature of practice as well as the intuitive intersections that can illuminate problems and sublimate the transformations that take place within practical research and the practice of research.

---

[22] Cited in John Pickles, *A History of Spaces: Cartographic Reason: Mapping and the Geo-Coded World* (New York: Routledge, 2004): 19.

WORKS CITED

Bhabha, Homi K. *The Location of Culture*. (London: Routledge, 1994).

Deleuze, Gilles, & Félix Guattari. *A Thousand Plateaus: Capitalism and Schizophrenia*, tr. Brian Massumi (*Capitalisme et schizophrénie* 2: *Mille plateaux*, 1980; Minneapolis: U of Minnesota P, 1986).

Derrida, Jacques, "The Time Before The First," in *The Derrida Reader: Writing Performances*, ed. Julian Wolfeys (Lincoln: U of Nebraska P, 1988): 130–39.

Dodge, Martin. "An Atlas of Cyberspaces," in *Cyber Geography Research* (2007), http://www.personalpagesmanchester.ac.uk (accessed 2008).

Fine, Michelle. "Working the Hyphens: Reinventing Self and Other in Qualitative Research," in *The Landscape of Qualitative Research: Theories and Issues*, ed. Norman K. Denizen & Yvonna S. Lincoln (Thousand Oaks CA: Sage, 1998): 130–55.

Foucault, Michel. "The Politics of Health in the Eighteenth Century" (1976), in *The Foucault Reader*, ed. Paul Rabinow (Harmondsworth: Penguin, 1984): 208–26.

Green, Paul. "Paul Baran and the Origins of the Internet," http://www.rand.org/about/history/baran.html (accessed 22 May 2010).

Kentridge, William. "The mouth of the crocodile," in *Ubu and the Truth Commission*, ed. Jane Taylor (Cape Town: U of Cape Town P, 1998): iii–xiv.

Macbeth, Douglas. "On 'reflexivity" in qualitative research: Two readings and a third," *Qualitative Inquiry* 7.1 (2001): 35–68.

Minh-ha, Trinh T. *The Digital Film Event* (London Routledge, 2005).

Moustakas, Clark. *Heuristic Research: Design, Methodology and Applications* (Thousand Oaks CA & London: Sage, 1990).

——. *Phenomenological Research Methods* (Thousand Oaks CA: Sage, 1994).

Myerhoff, Barbara, & Jay Ruby. "A Crack in a Mirror: Reflexive Perspectives in Anthropology," in *Remembered Lives: The Work of Ritual, Storytelling and Growing Older*, ed. Myerhoff & Marc Kaminsky (Ann Arbor: U of Michigan P, 1992): 307–40.

Nicholson, Helen. *Applied Drama: The Gift of Theatre* (New York: Palgrave Macmillan, 2005).

Pickles, John. *A History of Spaces: Cartographic Reason: Mapping and the Geo-Coded World* (New York: Routledge, 2004).

Schön, Donald. *The Reflective Practitioner: How Professionals Think in Action* (London: Temple Smith, 1983).

Steier, Frederick. *Research and Reflexivity* (Thousand Oaks CA: Sage, 1991).

Taylor, Victor E., & Charles Winquist. *Encyclopedia of Post Modernism* (New York: Routledge, 2001).

Yin, Robert K. *Case Study Research: Design and* Methods, vol. 5 (Thousand Oaks: Sage, 2003).

——. *Applications of Case Study Research*, vol. 34 (Thousand Oaks CA: Sage, 2003).

⌘

REMO CHIPATISO

Evaluation of Applied Drama and Theatre in HIV/AIDS Interventions

A Case Study of Themba Interactive

Introduction

A NUMBER OF SCHOLARS have written about how powerful drama and theatre are. As the teacher Michael Rodd points out,

> the theatre allows us to converse with our souls – to passionately pursue and discover ways of living with ourselves and others. We are all artists, and theatre is a language. We have no better way to work together, to learn about each other, to heal and to grow.[1]

Augusto Boal also asserts:

> theatre is born when the human being discovers that it can observe itself; when it discovers that, in this act of seeing, it can see *itself* – see itself *in situ*: see itself seeing. [...] A triad comes into being. The observing-I, the I-*in-situ*, and the not-I, that is, the other.[2]

These comments raise the question of *how* this is possible. Are drama and theatre not just mere entertainment which is inapplicable to developmental

---

[1] Michael Rodd, quoted in Philip Taylor, *Applied Theatre: Creating Transformative Encounters in the Community* (Portsmouth NH: Heinemann, 2003): xix.

[2] Augusto Boal, *The Rainbow of Desire: The Boa Method of Theatre and Therapy*, tr. Adrian Jackson (*O arco-íris do desejo: método Boal de teatro e terapia*, 1990; Abingdon & New York: Routledge, 1995): 13 ("Theatre, the First Human Invention").

projects? What positions drama and theatre as having the capacity to bring about transformation? Is this premise valid? If so, in what manner do drama and theatre achieve this? Is transformation of the complex human being truly attainable in a theatrical setting? What effect can applied drama and theatre have in HIV/AIDS interventions and developmental interventions generally?

In trying to respond to these questions, this essay explores the effectiveness of applied drama and theatre, using Themba Interactive as a case study.

Background of Themba Interactive

Themba Interactive is a Johannesburg-based non-governmental organization involved in using applied drama and theatre to address health and social issues, including HIV/AIDS, among youth and adults in South Africa. The organization was launched in February 2002 in Sophiatown. After nine years it has reached out to more than 70,000 South Africans, educating them about health and social issues, mainly HIV/AIDS, through interactive theatre. Themba Interactive trains its own actors and facilitators from disadvantaged backgrounds, constantly creating jobs for youth. It started as a project for school drop-outs in Alexandra Park and Soweto, based at the Trevor Huddleston Memorial Centre in Sophiatown, but has since grown to become a full-time organization with members drawn from various areas around Johannesburg and beyond. Themba Interactive was the winner of the *Mail and Guardian* Most Innovative Award in 2007, having been runner-up in 2006.

Themba Interactive is not only involved in interventions related to HIV/AIDS education, but takes a broader look at health and social issues that include sexual and gender-based violence, and sexual orientation, among many others. This essay, however, will focus on its HIV/AIDS programme. It provides participatory workshop performances under its Interactive Themba Theatre (ITT) wing, and training under its Themba Training Initiative (TTI) wing, for community-based organizations, schools, and correctional centres in South Africa. The workshop performances are aimed at addressing HIV/AIDS-related issues affecting communities by using role as the central aspect. The training is meant for the practitioners, who will then be able to work with communities in HIV/AIDS education.

The workshop performances are used to promote dialogue, thus at times serving as a stimulant to the follow-up training workshops. Themba Interactive is also a training organization for its actor–educators. Although the organization has managed to offer training and workshop performances in other provinces in South Africa, it has mainly catered to Gauteng province as its primary target. It may look as though there are two separate wings within Themba Interactive with separate staff; however, the organization has managed to train most of its staff to fit easily into either training or workshop-performance programmes. This means that they are able to perform their duties either in training under the TTI or in workshop performances under ITT.

This essay focuses on the workshop performances in the HIV/AIDS programme. In its workshop performances, Themba Interactive uses interactive theatre techniques from various drama and theatre forms such as forum theatre, dramatherapy, process drama, drama in education, psychodrama, and theatre for development. In order to closely analyse the Themba Interactive's work, role theory is used as the critical lens. Francis Nye points out that role theory is not one theory; rather, it is a set of concepts and interrelated theories that are at the foundation of social science in general.[3] Actions between persons are organized into roles and human conduct is the product of the interaction of the self and role. A role is a sequenced pattern of learned actions or deeds performed by a person in an interaction.[4] By performing a particular action in applied drama and theatre, participants undergo transformations and role becomes a source of epiphany (a moment of sudden understanding or revelation that occurs to an individual as a result of undergoing an experience).

The Modes of Communication in Interactive Themba Theatre

The significance of role in HIV/AIDS intervention lies in its ability to assist communication between the actor–educators and the spectators. Role stimulates interaction in an intervention, which is vital in the communication process. ITT uses the interactive approach, of which role is central, in order to ensure effective communication between the actor–educators and the spectators. This communication process takes many forms; it is not just verbal communication, but encompasses signs and symbols. According to Keir Elam,

---

[3] Francis Ivan Nye, *Role Structure and Analysis of the Family* (Thousand Oaks CA: Sage, 1976).

[4] Richard Courtney, *Play, Drama, and Thought: The Intellectual Background to Drama in Education* (London: Cassell & New York: Collier Macmillan, 1974): 227.

> An adequate account must be able to identify the range of sign repertories making up what might be termed the theatrical system or systems; to explain the internal (syntactic) relations of each and the interrelations between systems; and to make explicit the kinds of rules which allow meaning to be communicated and received in the performer–spectator dialectic.[5]

In HIV/AIDS education there is a need for a performer–spectator dialectic in order for the intervention to be beneficial to both parties.

It is the need for effective interaction between actor–educators and spectators in HIV/AIDS education that makes role so important in an intervention. This, as highlighted by Elam, is dependent on the relationships that can be observed in an intervention. Themba Interactive's work consists of modes of communication that make role significant in HIV/AIDS interventions. These are participatory, reflective, reversal, and reflexive modes. The presence of these modes of communication is important in HIV/AIDS education and also tend to operate in contexts of behavioural change. A number of interventions that have been previously carried out in communities overlooked the use of role, which is central to all theatre, in engaging with spectators. This essay examines the effectiveness of these modes of communication in ITT interventions.

Participatory Mode

Communication between the facilitators and the spectators in the early days of applied drama and theatre has been described in some theatre circles as a one-way communication system. Scholars such as Kerr, Kidd, Freire, Desai, and Boal have highlighted the challenges that occur in the communication process between facilitators and spectators in interventions.[6] These scholars assert the

---

[5] Keir Elam, *The Semiotics of Theatre and Drama* (London & New York: Methuen, 1980): 32.

[6] David Kerr, "Participatory Popular Theatre: The Highest Stage of Cultural Under-Development?," *Research in African Literatures* 22.3 (Fall 1991): 55–75; Ross Kidd, "Popular Theatre and Nonformal Education in the Third World: Five Strands of Experience," *International Review of Education* 30.3 (1984): 265–87; Paulo Freire, *Pedagogy of the Oppressed*, tr. Myra Bergman Ramos (*Pedagogía del oprimido*, 1971; tr. 1972; New York: Continuum, 1993); Gaurav Desai, "Introduction: Theatre for Development in Africa," *Research in African Literatures* 22.3 (Fall 1991): 6–10; Augusto Boal, *Theatre of the Oppressed*, tr. Charles A. McBride, María–Odilia Leal McBride & Emily Fryer (*Teatro do oprimido e outras poéticas políticas*, 1975; tr.1979;

need for a model that allows participation of both parties in an intervention. Jennings avers that "the model of development of a person lies in social interaction and transactions of the individual with others in an environment."[7] In ITT interventions, the participatory mode is the basis on which the process relies. The spectators' involvement is evident in their contribution and response to questioning, hot-seating, simultaneous dramaturgy, reflection, and role playing. Role as a central aspect of the intervention allows the actor–educators to interact with the spectators in a process where both parties are bound to benefit. It is this interaction that allows role to speak to both the actor–educators and the spectators through identification and projection.

HIV/AIDS education and behavioural change depends on the perception of the self. In order for there to be any development of the self, the intervention must accommodate that self in a participatory mode. The development of the self builds on the philosophy of symbolic interaction through role. As Cecily O'Neill points out,

> All forms of theatre, including improvised drama, have in common the need for an audience. The spectators and their participation in the encounter define it as theatre, which does not mean merely what the actors do in the presence of the audience. The spectators are essential in the realisation of the work and without them no theatre event is complete.[8]

The spectator's influence is necessary in applied drama and theatre. In the ITT interventions, spectator participation is vital, in that it shapes the intervention to a certain extent. The spectators are able to engage in questioning actor–educators and in making suggestions in a process similar to Boal's simultaneous dramaturgy. This enables role to be able to speak to the spectators via a participatory mode. The limitation in ITT interventions is that spectators' involvement is given limited time and the questions and suggestions tend to be guided. The spectators are shaped to react and act in positive ways.

New York: Theatre Communications Group, 1985), *Games for Actors and Non-Actors*, tr. Adrian Jackson (*200 exercícios e jogos para o ator e o não-ator com vontade de dizer algo através do teatro*, 1977; London: Routledge, 1992), and *The Rainbow of Desire*.

[7] Sue Jennings, Ann Cattanach, Steve Mitchell, Anna Chesner & Brenda Meldrum, *The Handbook of Dramatherapy* (London & New York: Routledge, 1994): 75.

[8] Cecily O'Neill, *In Drama Worlds: A Framework for Process Drama* (Portsmouth NH: Heinemann, 1995): 111.

This can result in pseudo-participation, as most spectators will adopt a prescribed positive attitude in the intervention, something that may be false and not what they would do in real life when dealing with HIV/AIDS.

Role creates dramatic worlds which allow the interaction of the performer and the spectator. Haseman and O'Toole assert:

> Working in drama involves stepping into an imagined world. To make this imaginary world of drama meaningful and purposeful, it must have aspects of the real world in it. The central, real world component of dramatic situations is human relationships.[9]

Through the use of role in the creation of dramatic worlds, ITT manages to engage with the spectators as active participants in the process. The performances are used to create imaginary worlds, with role-play as a mediating force in the presentation of the themes in order for the spectators to participate actively. By creating dramatic worlds, ITT is able to engage spectators in a way that allows them to come to terms with HIV/AIDS issues. HIV/AIDS is often associated with a range of psychological challenges which individuals, families, and communities struggle to come to terms with. HIV/AIDS has an impact on the infected and/or affected socially, emotionally, and psychologically. Through the use of role in the plays presented before them and also by being involved in role-playing, spectators are able to cope with their fears and emotions. By creating the dramatic worlds, a safe space is framed that allows the spectators to participate in the ITT interventions. The use of a prepared performance, however, has one potential weakness, in that it tends to result in the use of a 'one size fit all' approach where the same performance is used for various spectators. Dividing the spectators merely into youths and adults is not enough to address the complexity of HIV/AIDS.

Applied drama and theatre thrive when spectators are able to realize the need for their involvement. It operates from the awareness that there are issues in communities that need to be addressed, and participatory theatre is one way of dealing with them. The spectators need to be in a participatory mode, despite the fact that the intervention would have been initiated by external facilitators. The notions of participation and inclusivity enable people to take control of their lives, and are central principles in applied theatre. Philip Taylor points out that "there is an obligation in which audience members ob-

---

[9] Brad Haseman & John O'Toole, *Dramawise: An Introduction to the Elements of Drama* (Port Melbourne: Heinemann, 1986): 3.

serve a theatre presentation, or scenario, and also participate in it."[10] This is the case with ITT interventions. The spectators participate in a process that involves presenting a prepared play, which they then engage with in a participatory mode.

It is through participation that the spectators are able to at least come to terms with their problems. Boal's pedagogy does not deliver the finished product to its audience to be digested; if anything, it delivers a process, a provocation.[11] Through participation in the process, the spectators are able to go through an experience that is vital in coming to terms with the HIV/AIDS epidemic, rather than being told what to do. By becoming 'spect-actors' (active members as described by Boal) in the ITT interventions, the spectators are able to face their HIV/AIDS fears and emotions. It is this capacity of the spectators to become 'spect-actors', where they consciously and deliberately reflect and act on the implications of their own and other's actions, that is central to applied drama and theatre. This not only allows them to grapple with HIV/AIDS on a personal level but also gives them an understanding of others.

Role has to be motivated in order to engage the spectators in a participatory mode. John O'Toole argues that "a drama frames a particular set of interactive behaviours between people, each of whom has purposes and motivation towards goals."[12] Role motivation allows spectators to engage in a participatory mode. The roles in ITT interventions speak to spectators by bringing out the HIV/AIDS themes that they identify with. This allows them to step into the dramatic world and participate:

> The entire occurrence is a kind of conspiracy by both the watchers and the watched to establish and believe in the imaginary world that is being created and presented. Although it appears the actors are in control of this conspiracy, the audience can be regarded as the senior partner in this relationship, calling the tune, as it were, and even indirectly employing all those engaged in creating the theatrical experience.[13]

---

[10] Philip Taylor, *Applied Theatre: Creating Transformative Encounters in the Community*, 4.

[11] Adrian Jackson, "Translator's Introduction" to Boal, *The Rainbow of Desire*, xxiv.

[12] John O'Toole, *The Process of Drama: Negotiating Art Through Meaning* (London & New York: Routledge, 1992): 73.

[13] O'Neill, *In Drama Worlds: A Framework for Process Drama*, 112.

This type of experience demands active mediation by the spectators, who speculate, make assumptions, apply interpretations, and develop expectations about the make-believe world that is unfolding before them. It is through this interaction with role that the spectators engage in a participatory mode in the ITT interventions.

Taylor points out that "applied theatre works best when the participants are actively engaged, critically exploring the implications of their own and other's actions."[14] It is by engaging in a participatory mode that the spectators find meaning in the ITT interventions and come to terms with the HIV/AIDS epidemic through projection and identification. By agreeing to step into imaginary worlds where there is interaction between the role and the self, the spectators discover new lessons about HIV/AIDS. The participatory mode is vital in HIV/AIDS response programmes, as it engages the spectators in a process where their role-playing in a situation in workshop performance constitutes a rehearsal for real life. This puts them in the shoes of the other in an experience that allows role to interact with the self on HIV/AIDS-related issues. The ITT, however, needs to give more time to the spectators on the various levels of participation. Developing the spectators' trust and valuing their thoughts will result in better and more beneficial interventions rather than being perfunctory and failing to explore the challenges which some spectators are bound to raise. Going through a participatory mode that allows effective expression will prove to be vital in raising and addressing HIV/AIDS challenges.

Reflective mode

The reflection in applied drama and theatre involves finding meaning in the roles played in a fictional mode. Landy[15] points out that this helps in assessing the value of drama, validating feelings and providing needed translations from the world of imagination to that of the here and now, and from the contained dramatic space to the less controlled space of everyday life. The reflective mode enables the spectators in the ITT interventions to find meaning in the roles that are presented before them. Spectators are given space to be reflective and find the spectator–self in interventions in order for them to find meaning. It is the use of role as a central aspect in the ITT interventions that

---

[14] Taylor, *Applied Theatre: Creating Transformative Encounters in the Community*, 5.

[15] Robert Landy, *Persona and Performance: The Meaning of Role in Drama, Therapy, and Everyday Life* (New York & London: Guilford, 1993): 51.

emerges as a vital aspect providing room for the reflective mode for both actor–educators and spectators.

The reflective mode enables the spectators to be constantly in and out of the dramatic world. This involves interacting with the roles in the dramatic worlds and constantly finding the essences of that presentation in their everyday lives. The purpose and form of the roles in an intervention need to be clear for the spectators to be engaged in a reflective mode. In the ITT interventions, this is centred on how roles are played in bringing out the connection between feeling and thought. Roles in the ITT interventions have clear purposes, enabling the spectators to engage in a reflective mode. Getting in such a mode enables spectators to revisit their positions and thoughts on HIV/AIDS, and to try to find the best way to respond to HIV/AIDS on both family and community levels:

> When applied theatre operates well it can challenge audience members, spectators, to ask themselves questions: what might I do if I were placed in the same circumstances? How does the experience being demonstrated in front of me relate to my own life circumstances? To what extent can I learn from the experience? How might my life be changed or transformed?[16]

Of course, it is not always the case that applied drama and theatre achieve this state; there are times when spectators are merely entertained and not challenged to rethink a familiar situation or contemplate previously unconsidered ideas. This has been the challenge for early forms of applied drama which emphasized awareness, just to let people know about HIV/AIDS. This is not wrong, of course; but the current interventions need to engage participants on a level much more in line with current HIV/AIDS trends. Through the use of role, ITT enlists spectators in a reflective mode which permit better communication, which appeals to the self for spectators and actor–educators. The roles convey themes so as to enable spectators to identify or project within the intervention.

Through the presentation of roles before an audience in a dramatic world, ITT's actor–educators are able to enjoin spectators to reflect. This presentation invites the spectators to look at themselves in relation to the roles,, and by so doing they reflect upon themselves. As O'Neill points out,

> Anyone who publicly takes on a fictional role becomes at once both more and less than an individual. As soon as they are viewed as in

---

[16] Taylor, *Applied Theatre*, 6.

> even the most vestigial role actors require a corporeal exemplarity. Whether at the most developed end of the continuum of acting behaviour or at least personalised, actors represent different versions of humanity and will be recognised as types in a human family.[17]

Through identification and projection of themes via role-play, the spectators assess the value of the drama for their everyday lives. In the plays *Class of 2008* and *Heartbreaker* there are role personalities that spectators identify with and project from. This is important in that the play becomes a transformative agent that places the spectators in direct and immediate situations where they can witness, confront, and deconstruct aspects of their own and others' actions in relation to HIV/AIDS.

Reflection is vital in HIV/AIDS education if behavioural change is to be achieved. Engaging with the spectators in a reflective mode appeals to the self – an important element in influencing behavioural change. The centrality of role in ITT's cultivation of interactive process gives room for developing a reflective mode, not only for actor–educators but also for spectators. O'Neill asserts that playing the role is the means by which the very concept of role itself is investigated. In all kinds of drama, role-play is both the medium and the message upon which the reflective mode is based.[18] By using role, the ITT actor–educators manage to engage the spectators in a reflective mode.

ITT seeks to effect behavioural change among South Africans so that they engage in safer sex and live a healthy life-style. In order for ITT to achieve its purpose, spectators must be involved in a process of efficacy and transformation. This transformative principle shares a lot with other participatory and community-theatre movements, where a central emphasis is on the application of theatre to help people reflect more critically on the kind of society in which they live. Boal argues that at its most effective, theatre places audiences on both the inside and the outside of a virtual world,[19] and it is this duality that leads to significant reflective experiences. Freire confirms this:

> The heart of educational transformation is an enabling of human beings to consciously reflect on their actions and then change their behaviour in light of their discoveries. Such transformation is a praxis: action-reflection-transformation.[20]

---

[17] O'Neill, *In Drama Worlds: A Framework for Process Drama*, 70.

[18] *In Drama Worlds: A Framework for Process Drama*, 84.

[19] Boal, *Theatre of the Oppressed*, 3.

[20] In *Applied Theatre: Creating Transformative Encounters in the Community*, 9.

ITT, through its application of role-play, manages to a certain extent to engage the spectators in a reflective mode. The effectiveness could be more if the workshop performances give more time for reflection during and at the end of the intervention. If the reflective mode is to be a good model that benefits spectators in ITT, more room has to be provided for reflection to make it a better approach to HIV/AIDS interventions.

Reversal mode

Taking the role of the other in an intervention allows actor–educators and spectators to engage in a process where there is role-reversal. This involves taking the role of the other person in order to understand their feelings and thoughts. The ITT intervention gives room for this type of communication. According to Jennings et al., being in the role of another may give rise to a different set of behaviours and perhaps attitudes.[21] It is through role-reversal that spectators and actor–educators are able to interact in a process that will be beneficial to both parties, by engaging in mutual understanding of the roles presented.

Through role-reversal, spectators and actor–educators have an opportunity to interrogate the situation at hand:

> a participant 'steps into the shoes of another' in order to experience subjectively some aspects of that other, or the situation in which that other is found. To do that the subject must find the humanness of that other, acknowledging that he or she is capable of that other's actions and so identify with the character in the situation.[22]

People act and react differently in relation to HIV/AIDS. This arises from the fact that HIV/AIDS has psychological and emotional effects on the well-being of people, both the infected and the affected. It is the complexity of HIV/AIDS that gives role a place as one of the few meaningful ways through which people can come to understand each other.

In the ITT intervention, the actor–educators and the spectators engage in a reversal mode in order to make communication possible. During the 'breaking the silence' moment, spectators and actor–educators take turns playing the role of being HIV-positive, with the other part being that of a supportive friend. This, as indicated above, gives the spectators and the actor–educators

---

[21] Jennings et al., *The Handbook of Dramatherapy*, 75.

[22] O'Toole, *The Process of Drama: Negotiating Art Through Meaning*, 86.

an opportunity to feel what it's like to be in the shoes of the other. It is by going through this practical experience that the reversal mode enables communication between the infected and the uninfected. The challenge for ITT is that the spectators are told what to say as a response to an HIV-positive friend, it would be more effective if the spectator responded in a way they want. This would help ITT actor–educators find the problems that may exist among the participants, and then address them through role-play.

Power dynamics play a part in involving the spectators in interventions. If spectators are passive, there can be minimal benefits to them as compared to when they are actively involved. The reversal mode allows both the spectators and the actor–educators to take on active roles in the intervention. The existence of such a scenario results in a shared power relationship between spectator and actor–educators. Taylor asserts:

> Applied theatre pivots on the conviction that the theatre form can uniquely place individuals in situations where they can interrogate some issues, confront a problem, and analyse their relationship to the world in which they live.[23]

Through the reversal mode, spectators and actor–educators come to understand what it is like to be HIV-positive and what it is like to have AIDS. By understanding the feelings and thoughts of the other, issues such as HIV/AIDS stigma and discrimination can be tackled. Without a proper understanding of each other, the topic of HIV/AIDS can prove difficult to deal with. ITT's use of role-reversal helps engage the spectator in a mode that makes them face the reality of HIV/AIDS. The challenge for ITT interventions is that the spectators do not always express themselves but are, rather, told what to say at times. This may be of little benefit to spectators, since what they say will not be their own thoughts and feelings. Giving the spectators room for self expression could be more beneficial to ITT's work.

Understanding the consequences of our actions and the effects they have on others is very important. Jennings points out that "we know who we are through the way other people interact with us and reflect back to us the consequences of our behaviour towards them."[24] HIV/AIDS is a subject that requires one to be careful in relating to other people. It is through such interaction that the actor–educators and spectators engage in a reversal mode that

---

[23] Taylor, *Applied Theatre*, 4.

[24] Jennings et al., *The Handbook of Dramatherapy*, 82.

helps in HIV/AIDS communication. Through the reversal mode, embodiments of the whole dramatic situation can be invented, re-invented, and rearranged to allow spectators to experience what it is to be the other. In role-reversal, ITT spectators engage in an experience of discovery, thus rehearsing for life.

The reversal mode enables actor–educators and spectators to move from one state to the other in the dramatic encounter. The boundaries between the two sides become fluid, with room for engaging with and understanding the situation from both sides. The fluid boundaries allow the respective participants to learn who they are and what they could be in relation to HIV/AIDS. Looking at a situation from a different point of view is important when it comes to HIV/AIDS. The reversal mode in the ITT intervention offers a conducive environment for this to happen. It is the use of the reversal mode that enables actor–educators and spectators to reach a better understanding of one another, thus resulting in better ways of dealing with HIV/AIDS and its sensitivity as a subject.

Reflexive mode

The interaction of the self and role introduces an element of reflexiveness in the player of a role. Reflexiveness involves looking back at one self in the process of being engaged in an action. The ITT, through its use of role-play, manages to engage spectators in a reflexive mode through heightened involvement. The essential quality of the self is that it is reflexive;[25] we experience ourselves in the same way as we experience other objects and people. Responses to HIV/AIDS need to appeal to the human self in order to effect behavioural change. ITT focuses on the use of role in order to appeal to the self, engaging it in a process in which there is reflexiveness of oneself on HIV/AIDS issues.

Early interventions in applied drama and theatre under-emphasized the reflexive mode for the spectators, since they were not actively involved in role. The spectators were not present during role-creation and role-taking; they were even passive during the drama (role-play) and were only engaged after the drama. Involving spectators only in post-performance discussions is a disadvantage because it reduces participator involvement at all level of the intervention. Boal underscores the need for spectators to be actively involved in the action through taking on roles, not just participating from a seated posi-

---

[25] *The Handbook of Dramatherapy*, 81.

tion. It is through playing a role that reflexiveness can take place. In order for spectators to benefit from the interventions they have to take active roles in the process. However, ITT needs to give more time to spectators on role playing in the interventions in order to encourage self-reflexivity. Currently, few spectators get the opportunity to role-play, and this means self-reflexivity is limited to those individuals.

It is the level of active interaction between the self and the role that can allow self-reflexiveness. There are distinguishable levels of interaction between the self and the role in role-playing, from a point where there is consciousness to where there is unconsciousness, and these influence the mode of reflexivity.[26] The ITT interventions operate on a level where the self and the other consciously engage with each other. When this occurs successfully, it means that the role-player has room for self-reflexivity; "through the interaction of the self with the other, the self develops the ability to take on the perspectives of the other."[27] In HIV/AIDS' interventions there is a need to understanding others by role-playing in order to come to terms with the nature of HIV status. The interaction that occurs between the self and the role allows understanding of one another through self-reflexivity rather than being judgmental.

In the ITT interventions the spectators experience an event while controlling the nature of the experiences they are having. They engage in a form of internal dialogue in which they critique the experience at the very same moment in which they are submitting to that experience. When this occurs, the spectators are challenged to ask themselves such questions as 'What am I supposed to do in these circumstances?' This is the central aspect that needs to exist in HIV/AIDS intervention. Lack of understanding others affects HIV/AIDS response programmes. It is through empathetic coexistence that HIV/AIDS response programmes can be effective in addressing stigmatization. There has been 'othering' (polarization based on one's HIV status), and this has had a negative impact on campaigns so far. Society has been split into categories of the infected, the affected, and the uninfected. Through the use of role-play, which affords room for self-reflexivity,spectators in the ITT intervention engage in a process that can remove these barriers. At the end of the day we are all infected and/or affected by HIV/AIDS. In a play, *The Truth*

---

[26] See esp. Courtney, *Play, Drama, and Thought* passim.

[27] Jennings et al., *The Handbook of Dramatherapy*, 80.

About You, directed by Grace Meadows, othering is highlighted as one of the ways in which the HI virus thrives.

Role is a highly processual element in drama; of the various elements of drama, the metaxis between real and fictional contexts is most evident in role.[28] When spectators play a role they enter a liminal space which allows the interaction of the real and fictional worlds as "thought-in-action."[29] By engaging spectators in a liminal space, the intervention challenges participants to attempt a resolution in action. This is what makes the ITT intervention effective in the HIV/AIDS education process.

While applied drama and theatre can be a useful way for communities in crisis to express concerns about what is preventing them from reaching their aspirations; can outside interventionists really share the grief and devastation of these communities? When there is talk of transformation, whose transformations are being promoted and valued? This is a major challenge for applied drama and theatre. The challenge is certainly apparent when we investigate work that demands a huge emotional investment from the participants (actor–educators and spectators) such as HIV/AIDS education. This must not be merely about the spectators surrendering their capacity to think, rethink, and reflect on the nature of experiences they are having. The spectators must not merely experience but must actively contemplate and critique the nature of the experiencing. By using role-play in its reflexive mode, ITT enables spectator involvement in the intervention, ceding to them ownership of the process. The challenge, as earlier highlighted, is that only a few spectators experience that process and many are left out. Reducing the number of participants in an intervention and opening more space for role playing by spectators will enable more engagement for spectators through the reflexive mode.

Self-reflexivity is what makes the ITT interventions appeal to the spectator selves, as O'Neill concludes:

> Even the most limited and functional kind of role taking will demand some degree of self-transcendence, something that goes beyond the actual here and now. Participants in role play are simultaneously an audience to their own acts and observers of the consequences of these acts.[30]

---

[28] O'Toole, *The Process of Drama: Negotiating Art and Meaning*, 180.

[29] See the application of Boalian principles by Eugenio Barba, "Eurasian Theatre" (1982), *Tulane Drama Review* 32.3 (T119) (Fall 1988): 129.

[30] O'Neill, *In Drama Worlds: A Framework for Process Drama*, 80.

It is through such a utilization of role-play that the HIV/AIDS pandemic can be tackled. With the spectators going through this experience and getting to know the self and the other, a better understanding of HIV/AIDS can emerge in families and society at large.

Concluding Remarks

The best way of discovering ourselves and our powers and potentialities is through our encounter with others, both real and imaginary.[31] Through the dramatic roles and worlds that are available vicariously in theatre we can learn both who we are and what we may be. The participatory, reflective, reversal, and reflexive modes enable spectators to engage in the ITT interventions in ways that significantly promote to HIV/AIDS education. This also consolidates the 'interactiveness' of ITT's approach to engaging with the spectators on a level where they are able to explore the role, the self, and the other. Through the aforementioned modes the spectators move in and out of the dramatic projection. There is constant movement from the self in everyday life to the other in an imaginative dramatic world. This enables interaction between the real and dramatic world that is important for distancing emotional issues related to HIV/AIDS. As O'Neill concludes, "all great drama will work best by leaving much endowment of characters, place, and action to the audience."[32] Through these modes of communication, ITT gives spectators space to explore HIV/AIDS issues.

Works Cited

Barba, Eugenio. "Eurasian Theatre" (1982), *Tulane Drama Review* 32.3 (T119) (Fall 1988): 126–30.

Boal, Augusto. *Games for Actors and Non-Actors*, tr. Adrian Jackson (*200 exercícios e jogos para o ator e o não-ator com vontade de dizer algo através do teatro*, 1977; London: Routledge, 1992).

——. *The Rainbow of Desire: The Boal Method of Theatre and Therapy*, tr. Adrian Jackson (*O arco-íris do desejo: método Boal de teatro e terapia*, 1990; Abingdon & New York: Routledge: 1995).

[31] O'Neill, *In Drama Worlds: A Framework for Process Drama*, 91.

[32] *In Drama Worlds: A Framework for Process Drama*, 77.

——. *Theatre of the Oppressed*, tr. Charles A. McBride, María–Odilia Leal McBride & Emily Fryer (*Teatro do oprimido e outras poéticas políticas*, 1975; tr. 1979; New York: Theatre Communications Group, 1985).

Courtney, Richard. *Play, Drama, and Thought: The Intellectual background to Drama in Education* (London: Cassell & New York: Collier Macmillan, 1974).

Desai, Gaurav. "Introduction: Theatre for Development in Africa," *Research in African Literatures* 22.3 (Fall 1991): 6–10.

Elam, Keir. *The Semiotics of Theatre and Drama* (London & New York: Methuen, 1980).

Freire, Paulo. *Pedagogy of the Oppressed*, tr. Myra Bergman Ramos (*Pedagogía del oprimido*, 1971; tr. 1972; New York: Continuum, 1993).

Haseman, Brad, & John O'Toole. *Dramawise: An Introduction to the Elements of Drama* (Port Melbourne: Heinemann, 1986).

Jackson, Adrian. "Translator's Introduction" to Boal, *The Rainbow of Desire*, xviii–xxvi.

Jennings, Sue, Ann Cattanach, Steve Mitchell, Anna Chesner & Brenda Meldrum. *The Handbook of Dramatherapy* (London & New York: Routledge, 1994).

Kerr, David. "Participatory Popular Theatre: The Highest Stage of Cultural Under-Development?," *Research in African Literatures* 22.3 (Fall 1991): 55–75.

Kidd, Ross. "Popular Theatre and Nonformal Education in the Third World: Five Strands of Experience," *International Review of Education* 30.3 (1984): 265–87.

Landy, Robert. *Persona and Performance: The Meaning of Role in Drama, Therapy, and Everyday Life* (New York & London: Guilford, 1993).

Nye, Francis Ivan. *Role Structure and Analysis of the Family* (Thousand Oaks CA: Sage, 1976).

O'Neill, Cecily. *In Drama Worlds: A Framework for Process Drama* (Portsmouth NH: Heinemann, 1995).

O'Toole, John. *The Process of Drama: Negotiating Art Through Meaning* (London & New York: Routledge, 1992).

Taylor, Philip. *Applied Theatre: Creating Transformative Encounters in the Community* (Portsmouth NH: Heinemann, 2003).

Themba HIV/AIDS Organisation. *Annual Report* (Johannesburg, 2005).

⌘

TENDAI MTUKWA

Theatre as Border-Crossing Among Women Living with HIV

A Case Study of Zandspruit Informal Settlement

Introduction

THIS ESSAY DRAWS ON a theatre as therapy, education, and activism project that I facilitated with the Olive Leaf Foundation wellness programme in Johannesburg in 2009. The essay seeks to examine the extent to which the project enabled participants to cross the border between objectification and subjectivity. Prentki asserts that the primary principle of applied theatre is to enable participants to rediscover their innate capacities for play, for imagination, for creativity, and for relating to others by exploring the self in the other and the other in the self.[1]

In this essay, I will argue for applied theatre and how it can enable the crossing of the border between objectification and subjectivity. In the first part, I will outline the theoretical framework that was applied to frame the project under analysis. I will also provide a brief description of the process of the project in order to give the reader an idea of how it was conducted. I shall then show how the process attempted to enable participants to cross the border between objectification and subjectivity. In conclusion, I will examine whether the project was able to meet Prentki's principles of applied theatre.

---

[1] Tim Prentki, *The Applied Theatre Reader* (London: Routledge, 2009).

Brief Background of Project

Participants were members of the Olive Leaf Foundation, a wellness programme located in Zandspruit Informal Settlement about forty kilometres east of Johannesburg. In this project, I worked with a support group of women, all of whom were living with HIV. These women had been meeting regularly to receive informal education on healthy positive living, reproductive health, sexual responsibility and protection, and treatment adherence.

The objectives of this project were based on what I had set out to achieve as an applied-theatre scholar. Had I learnt enough to remove applied theatre from institutional classrooms and practise it meaningfully in the real world? I wanted to examine whether Prentki's principles of applied theatre could come to life and actually make a difference in real peoples' lives. I also wanted to test Henry Giroux's border pedagogy[2] against Prentki's principles of applied theatre. Giroux's understanding of border pedagogy centres on the thesis that it is when human beings gain new experiences and move away from their everyday ways of experiencing life that they can transform themselves.

Focus

The essay focuses particularly on how people can make use of theatre as a way of empowering themselves within their daily struggles – in this case, the daily challenges of women living with HIV in a squatter settlement. The project aimed at looking for ways in which applied theatre can give people tools for examining and understanding themselves and others.

The participants were twelve women, whose number always fluctuated. This was because not all participants came at all times. The women came to attend the workshops together with their infant children, mainly because the women reported that they were the basic carers for the latter, most of whom were under twelve months old and could not be left at home. Although the aim of the project was to focus solely on the women, the little children's presence could not be ignored. The children had to be recognized and appreciated, as they, too, reacted to the energy and activities within the project space and became an integral part of that process.

---

[2] Henry A. Giroux, *Border Crossing: Cultural Workers and the Politics of Education* (New York: Chapman & Hall, 1992).

Theoretical Framework: Applied Theatre as Border-Crossing Pedagogy

The study was informed by the fundamentals of border pedagogy as set forth by Giroux, according to whom border-crossing from the self to the other requires that participants experience the opportunity for new subject-positions, identities, and social relations. Giroux asserts that critical learning involves a re-understanding of everyday practices, with the objective of understanding the self, others, and the environment.

In this project there was a need for participants to find a way to re-engage with the grand narratives of their lives in order to understand them and construct a new and different version of themselves.

Border-crossing politics requires that the teacher–student relationship be re-defined in ways that allow students to draw upon their own personal experiences as real knowledge. This involves giving students the opportunity to not only speak but also engage critically with the grand narratives – hegemonic narratives that have come to be identified as the norm.

Border-crossing in this case required participants to locate themselves within the idea of positive living. The project needed participants to become subjects in the construction of their own identities within a wider community. There was a great need, therefore, to offer an opportunity for participants to express their feelings about different ideologies functional in their everyday life. This would give them a way of reconstructing their lives in the community.

Preliminary Findings

A basic principle of applied theatre is knowledge of one's target group in order to plan an effective intervention. Every little detail I could find out about the group became of the utmost importance. I needed to know the group's current challenges and their perceived desires as far as their lives were concerned. I needed to know what they wanted to do or change as people living positively.

I discovered that the participants had no previous experience of theatre. They stressed that they were not looking forward to any theatrical performances, as they considered themselves incapable of performing or acting. The mention of drama made participants very shy and wary; they drew back. The acceptable dress code for participants also meant that only certain kinds of interaction were possible. Most wore dresses and skirts, which meant that more physical and active exercises would be limited. The available working space (a truck container) was very limited and this further curtailed the kinds of games and warm-up exercises that could be used. Games that called for running around could not be played.

It is from these findings that I designed an applied-theatre plan with techniques to suit the participants and their needs.

Challenges

My first challenge: I had assumed that such techniques as theatre games, image theatre, and forum theatre[3] are simple to play. However, I soon discovered that these techniques were not so easy as I thought for participants to follow. Theatre games failed to initiate the interaction that I had expected. There was a sudden need to revise my implementation plan in order to find new ways of creating meaningful interaction with the group.

Secondly, as Blatner purports, we should not underestimate the prevalence of personal and cultural factors that operate to inhibit theatre performance, enactment, and expressing oneself in front of other people. Blatner maintains that such inhibitions become automatic, habitual, and unconscious.[4] Eleanor Irwin calls these psychic inhibitions to play.[5]

Finally, I soon realized I had entered into this community with what Ira Shor terms "zero paradigms"[6] – regarding participants as unknowing, needing

---

[3] Augusto Boal, *Theatre of the Oppressed*, tr. Charles A. McBride, María–Odilia Leal McBride & Emily Fryer (*Teatro do oprimido e outras poéticas políticas*, 1975; tr. 1979; London: Pluto, 2008).

[4] Adam Blatner, "Webpage Supplement: Inhibitions and Resistances to Drama" (20 September 2006). online supplement to Blatner, "Introduction" to *Interactive and Improvisational Drama: Varieties of Applied Theatre and Performance*, ed. Adam Blatner with Daniel J. Wiener, foreword by David Shepherd (Lincoln NE: iUniverse, 2007), www.interactiveimprov.com/inhibitions2drama.html (accessed 3 December 2013).

[5] Eleanor Irwin, "Psychoanalytic Approach to Drama Therapy," in *Current Approaches in Drama Therapy*, ed. Penny Lewis & David Read Johnson (2000; Springfield IL: Charles C. Thomas, 2nd ed. 2009): 240.

[6] Ira Shor, *Empowering Education: Critical Teaching for Social Change* (Chicago: U of Chicago P, 2009).

to be filled with knowledge, skills, facts, and ignoring the culture the participants bring into the space. I discovered that I had entered into this space with some preconceived notions from my own personal experiences in applied-theatre work.

Even as I explained my theatre games and demonstrated how to play them, no one was willing to accept my invitation to play. Participants simply watched me and could not join in the play. I became aware of my assumptions and remembered that participants were the masters of their own challenges – I had to put participants at the forefront of the experience. Participants had to find solutions to their challenges and choose what they wanted to do; they had to become what Gramsci terms organic intellectuals.[7]

All these challenges and assumptions aided me into re-working a new plan of action that would work for participants and meet their needs.

Project Analysis

Our following sessions would start with a song and a prayer, as the participants later suggested; this had been the group culture before I came to work with them and was observed at all sessions. It was my attempt to replace zero paradigms with critical paradigms that recognize the cultural background of participants in order to create better relationships between educators and students. As Shor asserts, educators need to allow students to bring in their culture and use it as a starting point to learning and teaching. The song and prayer provided a crossing of the border between art and reality – a calming way of entering into the world of theatre.

Warm-up games in the sessions played an important role in preparing participants for deeper processes to take place; these games provided a way for participants to move from one way of being and cross to being another. The real root of drama is make-believe play, a lively imaginative interactive process that most people wish they could recapture.[8] In theatre games, partici-

[7] Antonio Gramsci, *Selections from the Prison Notebooks* (London: Lawrence & Wishart, 1971).

[8] Adam Blatner & Allee Blatner, *The Art of Play: An Adult's Guide to Imagination and Spontaneity* (New York: Human Sciences, 1988): 50, 75, and "Role Exploration and Cognitive Flexibility," in *Sociodrama: Who's in Your Shoes?*, ed. Patricia Sternberg & Antonina Garcia, foreword by Zerka T. Moreno (Westport CT: Praeger, 2000): 232 (232–38).

pants gradually opened up to 'recapturing play', thereby opening themselves up for something to take place.

During initial sessions, participants were satisfied by watching the 'other'. At first no participants were willing to join me in the games, even though I had explained and demonstrated these games. It seemed as if they were satisfied just to watch me play. Participants needed more convincing, further than just demonstrating, that it was safe to feel free, to be oneself and to enjoy play.

I continued to play alone in the space until interest was sparked in some participants; who then volunteered to join me in the space. Emunah and Johnson refer to this experience as the facilitator becoming the play-object.[9] As I continued to play, I showed participants that it was safe to do so. Jean–Paul Sartre asserts that we experience ourselves as an object in relation to others;[10] we come to know ourselves because of others and our experiences with them. Games managed to make participants see themselves in the other and to convince them to cross the border and join in.

Theatre games not only loosened muscles; something inside was also loosened. Participants began to look at themselves in different ways. They began to enjoy themselves. As we played on, participants soon became animated, with lots of laughter at themselves and their friends as they played along. Some of the children saw their mothers laughing and moving about the room, and themselves joined in the play and laughter within the aesthetic space.

One participant confessed that the games made her realize she had not been laughing recently, but had begun doing so a lot more both within and (importantly) beyond the space since she started attending the sessions. She disclosed that this was why she had invited some of her friends to come and partake in this enjoyment even when they were not members of the OliveLeaf wellness programme.

The fact that initial applied-drama techniques failed to have an impact on the group required that new borders be crossed by participants. Some participants did not have the confidence to get up in front of their colleagues to join in any activity. This led to an agreement among participants to do something to help those who were too shy. One woman reported that she felt so shy

---

[9] René Emunah & David Read Johnson, "The Current State of the Field of Drama Therapy," in *Current Approaches in Drama Therapy*, ed. Lewis & Johnson, 28.

[10] Discussed by Johnson in "Developmental Transformations: Towards the Body as Presence," in *Current Approaches in Drama Therapy*, 92.

about 'acting' in front of others that she needed some practice. There was thus a need for confidence-building in order to play basic theatre games and be able to continue. It was agreed to build a role repertoire as a way of gaining the skills the group needed. Role repertoire in this case meant building basic confidence skills through elementary role-playing. In this activity, participants were required to identify familiar roles, create short scenarios and find scene objectives, and comment on each others' role-playing skills. From my observations and to judge from their reports, this turned out to be an enjoyable exercise.

Through the games and exercises, applied theatre attempted to offer participants a chance to embrace and personify power. This produced 'activists' within the space, in the sense that it was practical and required participants to get up and be active. As Boal maintains, empowerment takes place within the body, on which language and action have an effect.[11] Power was rehearsed and practised within the body in the performance space, which translated into what Boal refers to as the "rehearsal for a revolution."[12]

This activism in practice through role-playing and theatre games resulted in major breakthroughs for some participants. After playing a version of *Madam and Eve*,[13] one member of the group reported having enjoyed playing the powerful Madam. Her willingness to try out and play a powerful, harsh, and unforgiving woman was a way of experiencing power outside of her usual self, thereby gaining new experiences.

Nevertheless, one member of the group was unable to embrace this power. This was cause for much agitation on the part of other members who saw this, rather, as an opportunity to practise power. One may argue that her knowledge of life had conditioned her to submission. This participant needed to be gently aided to cross the border of her fears until she managed to embody power. In the case of most other participants, powerful roles were more appreciated than the weaker ones. This suggests that the aesthetic space offered an

---

[11] Augusto Boal, *Games for Actors and Non-Actors*, tr. Adrian Jackson (*200 exercícios e jogos para o ator e o não-ator com vontade de dizer algo através do teatro*, 1977; London: Routledge, 1992): passim.

[12] Boal, *Games for Actors and Non-Actors*, 155.

[13] *Madame and Eve* is a daily cartoon strip by Stephen Francis and Rico Schacherl which satirizes the power dynamics between female householders and their maids in South Africa.

safe, alternative space in which to experience power without consequences. The aesthetic space offered alternatives to everyday experiences.

Bernie DeKoven maintains that theatre games are theatre itself, that playing is in fact drama. Dramatic play offered a space to practise spontaneity, which is a necessary activity for vitality and a healing tool.[14] As they played, participants were challenged to question general beliefs about playing games as adults in a community where, they confessed, adult play was not the norm.

Dramatic play helped to relieve different forms of anxiety. I soon observed that playing provided an intense absorption arising from the fun, which seemed to wield the power to move participants to another, joyful state of being.

Applied theatre worked to remove passivity and encouraged initiative, interaction, and collaboration. The major index of this was the fact that participants were able to think of the future of their activities. When it appeared that the project would soon end, participants became concerned. The women came up with a plan for how to continue their activities beyond the duration of the project. They were inspired by the significance of their work, such that they wanted to remain involved. They requested a copy of the theatre games and exercises that I had worked through with them so that they could use them in the future. This suggests a new sense of independence and the freedom to choose what they wanted to do for themselves in the future – an awakened awareness of the power and rewards of creativity.

In this case, theatre managed to offer a platform for a dual effect to take place, where art overlapped or intertwined with reality, creating a space called metaxis. According to Vygotsky's dual effect, social interaction plays a fundamental role in development and cognition.[15] During the process of dual effect, participants were able to connect with themselves and think of the future. Thus, from the experiences of play came an awakening to do something in their real lives.

In the light of this new consciousness, '*bophilong*' became the general theme for most sessions that went on after this initial suggestion of continuity. Participants explained to me the meaning of the word and how they found

---

[14] Bernie DeKoven, "Theater of Games," in *Interactive and Improvisational Drama*, ed. Blatner, 332 (332–40).

[15] Lev Semenovich Vygotsky, "Play and its Role in the Mental Development of the Child" (1933), http://www.marxists.org/archive/vygotsky/works/1933/play.htm (accessed 20 June 2010).

meaning and relevance for the word within the theatre space. *Bophilong* can be translated as 'a place of life'. After much debate among themselves, participants finally agreed on the theme of *bophilong* for continuity. This came up because participants regarded the aesthetic space as a site in which some had gained a rekindled awareness of life.

As sessions continued, participants began to open up even deeper issues that went beyond the objectives of the project. One much older participant began to reflect on the hardships experienced during the pre-independence, apartheid era. This can be an indication that the theatre space had become a safe, trusted, aesthetic space where participants felt they could unpack issues that were not normally discussed in their daily lives.

Arguably, participants had come a long way; applied theatre had helped them to be bolder than they had been initially. Initially shy and inactive, they now took a lead in discussions of issues within the group. The changes taking place within the space went beyond the ludic and enabled participants to reflect on deeper life issues. O'Connor maintains that the gap between the performer self and the audience self involves both the fictional and the real.[16] This gives an opportunity for reflection about whom and what we are as human beings.

Participants reflected on how attending sessions provided them with a form of relief and a place in which to relax from their daily challenges. The activity of reflection and 'de-roling'[17] functioned to move participants out of the imaginary, leaving the fictional behind. This was aimed at creating critical distance from the events of the project. Freire asserts that when men and women reflect on themselves, they increase the scope of their perception. They begin to direct their observations to 'previously inconspicuous pheno-

---

[16] Peter J. O'Connor, "Reflection and Refraction: The Dimpled Mirror of Process Drama: How Process Drama Assists People to Reflect on Their Attitudes and Behaviours Associated with Mental Illness" (doctoral dissertation, Griffith University, Brisbane, 2003): 43 (paraphrasing David Booth, "Imaginary Gardens with Real Toads," *NADIE Journal* 14.2 [1990]: 23–25).

[17] For an explanation of this term in the sense of 'warming down' by getting back out of a negative role without adverse effects, see, for example, Anne Ancelin Schützenberger, "Transgenerational analysis and psychodrama: Applying and extending Moreno's concepts of the co-unconscious and the social atom to transgenerational links," in *Psychodrama: Advances in Theory and Practice*, ed. Clark Baim, Jorge Burmeister & Manuela Maciel (Hove & New York: Routledge, 2007): 169.

mena."[18] The process of reflecting on their activities thus provided participants with a chance to know what new insights they had gained.

Conclusion

Findings from this study show that drama has the ability to offer people a platform to observe themselves. This platform was an empowering and liberating space in which participants could become an 'other', embodying power and allowing them to move towards healing. The aesthetic space offered by applied theatre managed, to a greater extent than with some other techniques, to influence participants' perception of themselves and what they can do in their lives.

Prentki's principles for applied theatre became a vehicle for achieving Giroux's border-crossing among participants. The essence of laughter, fun, enjoyment, and celebration provided the players with unusual access to a fundamental component of their lives. They were able to see themselves and others in a new light. Applied theatre provided a space in which participants rediscovered themselves and their abilities.

WORKS CITED

Blatner, Adam. "Webpage Supplement: Inhibitions and Resistances to Drama" (20 September 2006). online supplement to Blatner, "Introduction" to *Interactive and Improvisational Drama: Varieties of Applied Theatre and Performance*, ed. Adam Blatner with Daniel J. Wiener, foreword by David Shepherd (Lincoln NE: iUniverse, 2007), www.interactiveimprov.com/inhibitions2drama.html (accessed 3 December 2013).

——, & Allee Blatner. *The Art of Play: An Adult's Guide to Imagination and Spontaneity* (New York: Human Sciences, 1988).

——. "Role Exploration and Cognitive Flexibility," in *Sociodrama: Who's in Your Shoes?*, ed. Patricia Sternberg & Antonina Garcia, foreword by Zerka T. Moreno (Westport CT: Praeger, 2000): 232–38.

Boal, Augusto. *Games for Actors and Non-Actors*, tr. Adrian Jackson (*200 exercícios e jogos para o ator e o não-ator com vontade de dizer algo através do teatro*, 1977; London: Routledge, 1992).

---

[18] Paulo Freire, *Pedagogy of the Oppressed*, tr. Myra Bergman Ramos (*Pedagogía del oprimido*, 1971; New York: Herder & Herder, 1972): 63.

——. *Theatre of the Oppressed*, tr. Charles A. McBride, María–Odilia Leal McBride & Emily Fryer (*Teatro do oprimido e outras poéticas políticas*, 1975; tr. 1979; London: Pluto, 2008).

Booth, David. "Imaginary Gardens with Real Toads," *NADIE Journal* 14.2 (1990): 23–25.

DeKoven, Bernie. "Theater of Games," in *Interactive and Improvisational Drama: Varieties of Applied Theatre and Performance*, ed. Adam Blatner with Daniel J. Wiener, foreword by David Shepherd (Lincoln NE: iUniverse, 2007): 332–40.

Emunah, René, & David Read Johnson. "The Current State of the Field of Drama Therapy," in *Current Approaches in Drama Therapy*, ed. Penny Lewis & David Read Johnson (2000; Springfield IL: Charles C. Thomas, 2nd ed. 2009): 24–36.

Freire, Paulo. *Pedagogy of the Oppressed*, tr. Myra Bergman Ramos (*Pedagogía del oprimido*, 1971; tr. 1972; New York: Herder & Herder, 1972).

Giroux, Henry A. *Border Crossing: Cultural Workers and the Politics of Education* (New York: Chapman & Hall, 1992).

Gramsci, Antonio. *Selections from the Prison Notebooks* (London: Lawrence & Wishart, 1971).

Irwin, Eleanor. "Psychoanalytic Approach to Drama Therapy," in *Current Approaches in Drama Therapy*, ed. Penny Lewis & David Read Johnson (2000; Springfield IL: Charles C. Thomas, 2nd ed. 2009): 235–51.

Johnson, David Read. "Developmental Transformations: Towards the Body as Presence," in *Current Approaches in Drama Therapy*, ed. Penny Lewis & David Read Johnson (2000; Springfield IL: Charles C. Thomas, 2nd ed. 2009): 89–116.

O'Connor, Peter J. "Reflection and Refraction: The Dimpled Mirror of Process Drama: How Process Drama Assists People to Reflect on Their Attitudes and Behaviours Associated with Mental Illness" (doctoral dissertation, Griffith University, Brisbane, 2003).

Prentki, Tim. *The Applied Theatre Reader* (London: Routledge, 2009).

Schützenberger, Anne Ancelin. "Transgenerational analysis and psychodrama: Applying and extending Moreno's concepts of the co-unconscious and the social atom to transgenerational links," in *Psychodrama: Advances in Theory and Practice*, ed. Clark Baim, Jorge Burmeister & Manuela Maciel (Hove & New York: Routledge, 2007): 155–74.

Shor, Ira. *Empowering Education: Critical Teaching for Social Change* (Chicago: U of Chicago P, 2009).

Vygotsky, Lev Semenovich. "Play and its Role in the Mental Development of the Child" (1933), http://www.marxists.org/archive/vygotsky/works/1933/play.htm (accessed 20 June 2010).

⌘

Notes on Contributors

HAZEL BARNES is a retired Head of Drama and Performance Studies at the University of KwaZulu–Natal, where she is a Senior Research Associate. She has been a Mellon Visiting Scholar to the University of Cape Town and is a member of the Management Committee and Chair of the Research Committee of Drama for Life, Division of Dramatic Arts, School of Arts, University of the Witwatersrand. Her research interests lie in the field of Applied Drama in which she has published a number of papers on drama and theatre applied to interculturalism and post-traumatic stress. She has also published on South African playwrights, in particular Greig Coetzee and Mandla Mbothwe.

GORDON BILBROUGH is the Financial Director and resident script writer for arrep: Theatre for Life. During the nineteen years he has been with arrep he has become interested in researching its methodology and effectiveness. Prior to this he has worked with a number of theatrical organizations such as PACT, Out of the Box, and Colin Law Productions.

GALIA BONEH is southern regional consultant and coordinator for performing arts studies at the Karev Foundation for Enrichment in Education in Israel. She holds a PhD in Culture and Performance from UCLA'S Department of World Arts and Cultures. Boneh has been studying, travelling and working in Africa for the past 15 years, and has specialized in HIV/AIDS and arts for the past 5 years under the guidance of Prof. David Gere. She has created popular performance in active response to the HIV/AIDS epidemic in collaboration with Iddi Saaka in Ghana (2006) and Malawi (2008), where they led the CHANCO-UCLA Performance Project.

KENNEDY CHINYOWA is Head of the Division of Dramatic Arts at the University of Witwatersrand. He has taught at several universities including the University of Zimbabwe, Griffith University (Australia), and the University of KwaZulu–Natal. He was a visiting scholar at the Centre for Applied Theatre Research at Griffith University where he obtained his PhD degree in Theatre for Development. He has won numerous research awards and has published widely in books and refereed journals.

REMO CHIPATISO has a Masters degree from the Drama for Life Programme and works with Themba Interactive. He has previously worked for Zimbabwe Television before, in 2005, joining Theory X Media, where he worked at management and performance/facilitation level. He was also on the Harare International Festival of Arts workshop facilitator panel for two years in 2006 and 2007.

NEHEMIAH CHIVANDIKWA teaches applied drama, acting, playmaking and performance at the University of Zimbabwe. His research interests include participatory theatre, gender and performance, design, educational theatre and theatre as empowerment. He has been involved in practical applied-theatre projects on disability and empowerment, theatre and democracy, conflict resolution, ethnic prejudice and women in law. He is currently writing a PhD on *Disability, participation and empowerment in Theatre for Development.*

DAVID KERR has taught Theatre and Media Studies at the Universities of Botswana, Malawi, and Zambia for over thirty years. He has also been involved in many NGO communication projects, particularly on social and human rights in Africa, Asia and Europe. Hi sbooks include *African Popular Theatre* and *Dance, Media Entertainment and Popular Theatre in South East Africa.* He is currently working on a manual on using theatre for communication about HIV/AIDS, and a research project about Media Ownership in Botswana.

JAMIE LACHMAN is the founder and director of Clowns without Borders – South Africa, a humanitarian organization that provides psycho-social support through laughter and play to communities affected by trauma in Southern Africa. Their intervention programmes combines clown performance, theatre arts education and mindfulness based training. Clowns without Borders has worked with over 150,000 participants in South Africa, Lesotho**Fehler! Textmarke nicht definiert.**, and Swaziland, and is currently developing local capacities for intervention. Lachman is a graduate of Yale University and the Dell'Arte International School for Physical Theatre.

PATRICK MANGENI is an academic, a poet and a playwright. He won a grant as Poet in Residence at Akademie Schloss Solitude in Stuttgart in 1996 and was guest poet at the 2003 Queensland Poetry Festival. He was also a featured writer at the 2005 Brisbane Writers Festival. His plays, *Operation Mulungusi* and *The Prince,* won the National Book Trust of Uganda Award in 2000. In addition he has published a children's novel, *The Great Temptation.* He lectures at the University of Uganda.

SELLOANE MOKUKU is a Drama for Life alumni and currently consultant for national regional and international organizations using applied drama and theatre processes to address HIV prevention among young people and adolescents as well as most at risk populations (MARP), particularly sex workers. She is a director of Liatla Productions, an independent productions company that specializes in social behaviour change.

TENDAI MTUKWA has an MA in Dramatic Art from Wits University. Her areas of interest include theatre for cultural communication, theatre for therapy, activism and education. She is passionate about using theatre for healing and transformation especially within the context of HIV/AIDS. She has performed at various festivals including the Harare International Festival of the Arts.

REBECCA ANN RUGG is Associate Chair of Playwriting at Yale School of Drama and was previously Director of New Projects and Dramaturg at the Joseph Papp/New York Theatre Festival. She has a particular interest in contemporary US playwriting, art and activism. Her translation of Serbian playwright Biljana Srbljanovic's *Family Stories* was produced at the Market Theatre, Cambridge Massachusetts, and was published in *American Theater,* April 2003.

EMELDA NGUFOR SAMBA lectures at the University of Yaounde 1, Cameroon, and is artistic director of the National Association of Theatre Troupes in Cameroon and co-ordinator of the Fobang Mundi Theatre, which uses theatre to disseminate health messages. She is a well-known Theatre for Development consultant as well as an actress. She was part of the International Visitors Program on Performing Arts in the USA in 2005, and has conducted numerous training of trainers workshops in the area of theatre for social change in Cameroon and Germany.

ALEXANDRA SUTHERLAND lectures in the Drama Studies Department at Rhodes University, Grahamstown, South Africa where she specializes in applied-theatre theory and practice. She is the founder of the Art of the Street project, a youth theatre initiative for street and shelter based young people, and has worked (often with students) on numerous applied-theatre projects, including theatre in prisons, theatre and science and health education, theatre and heritage initiatives, and more recently, the use of theatre to examine issues of race, gender, class, and HIV in higher education.

MYER TAUB is a research fellow at the Research Centre for Visual Identities and Design, University of Johannesburg. He was recently awarded an interdisciplinary arts residency at The Bag Factory artist studio Fordsburg where he has thus far created two projects for them centred around urban interventions, video and performance. He has a PhD in Drama from the University of Cape Town.

JOHANNES VISSER has taught and lectured at various institutions before joining the staff of Drama at the University of Pretoria. Professional and training activities include directing, writing and facilitating over fifty theatre and educational productions. Current research includes applied theatre, the use of improvisation in actor training, and cultural and eco-tourism.

DIANA WILSON AND KAREN SUTER both work at the University of KwaZulu–Natal. Diana Wilson has worked as a professional actress, lectured, and directed and trained actors at the Drama Studio, London. She has also worked in education in Zimbabwe.

Karen Suter has worked as a production manager and currently as administrator of Drama and Performance Studies. They jointly devised and coordinated *The Lover and Another* Performance Poetry Competition.

⌘

Onomastic Index

AAA-HA! (Applied Arts for HIV/AIDS Awareness) 127, 132, 139
Abah, Oga S. 13
ACTUP New York 86
African Medical Research Foundation 213
Ahmed, Syed Jamil 206
AIDS Coalition to Unleash Power 86
Alexandra Park (SA) 252
Amakhosi Theatre (Zimbabwe) 207, 212
AMREF (African Medical Research Foundation) 213
Applied Arts for HIV/AIDS Awareness (AAA-HA!) 127, 132, 139
Archimedes 146
arepp: Theatre for Life 61–80
Aristotle and theatre 32
Arnold, David 180
ArtAction 221
Asetena pa Project (Ghana) 187
Ashcroft, Bill, Gareth Griffiths & Helen Tiffin 213
Asinamali (Mbongeni) 34
Atherton, James S. 64

Bakayimbira Dramactors 6, 29
Balfour, Michael 166, 206
Balme, Christopher 210, 211
Bangladesh 9
Baran, Paul 239
Barba, Eugenio 265
Beauvoir, Simone de 148
Bee, Francis, & Roland Bee 155, 158
Benjamin, Walter 32, 183
Bernard Van Leer Foundation 223
Bhabha, Homi K. 239
Bharucha, Rustom 211
Bilbrough, Gordon 62, 67, 69, 71, 72
Blantyre (Malawi) 33
Blatner, Adam 272, 273, 276; & Allee Blatner 273
Boal, Augusto 35, 53, 54, 55, 57, 84, 149, 150, 158, 162, 251, 254, 255, 257, 260, 263, 265, 272, 275; *Games for Actors and Non-Actors* 255, 275; *Legislative Theatre* 84; *The Rainbow of Desire* 251, 255, 257; *Theatre of the Oppressed* 53, 54, 55, 149, 150, 158, 254, 260, 272
Bogart, Anne 53
Booth, David 277
Booyens, Karen 166
Botswana xiii, 31, 35, 36, 37, 38, 212
Boud, David 65
Bourgault, Louise 181
British Council 49

British Council InterAction Leadership Programme 49
Buganda 25
Bulawayo 207
Butler, Judith 148

Cameroon xiii, 58–59
Campbell, Catherine 190, 191
Canadian International Development Agency 221
Cape Town 62, 67, 68, 69, 79, 80, 82, 91, 235–49
Center for Art | Global Health (UCLA) 187
Centre for AIDS Development Research 213
Centre for the Rehabilitation of the Disabled (Yaounde) 58
Chachage, Charles 120
Chambers, Robert 205, 209
Chameleon, Jose 18
Chancellor College (University of Malawi) 188, 199
CHANCO-UCLA Performance Project 188, 194, 196, 199
Chewa people (Malawi) 206
Chifunyise, Stephen 32
Chinyowa, Kennedy 212
Churchill, Winston 165
Clowns Without Borders 83, 85, 103, 104, 169, 220, 221, 222, 224, 225, 226, 231, 232
C-Max prison (Pretoria) xvi, 161, 162, 167
Coleman, Peter T. 214
Coleman–Tobias, Meredith 87, 92, 104, 106
Communication for Development Group (FAO) 206
Compaine, Benjamin M., & Douglas Gongery 33
Cooperrider, David L., & Diana Whitney 49, 51, 53, 54, 56, 59
Coplan, David 210
Courtney, Richard 253, 264
Croatia 220
CSA (Centre for the Study of AIDS, Pretoria) 161, 162, 166, 169, 172
CWB (Clowns Without Borders) 83, 85, 103, 104, 169, 220, 221, 222, 224, 225, 226, 231, 232
CWBSA artists collective (South Africa) 103, 104, 106, 220, 221, 222, 223, 227, 228, 229, 230, 231

Dalrymple, Lynn 62, 207, 212; & Paul Botha 207
Darder, Antonia, Marta Baltodano & Rodolfo Torres 205
Deacon, Harriet 180
DeKoven, Bernie 276
Deleuze, Gilles, & Félix Guattari 240, 249
Dempster, Carolyn 164, 165
Derrida, Jacques 238
Desai, Gaurav 254
Dewey, John 63, 65
Dey, Ian 67
Dick, Bob 62, 63
Disability Resource Centre (Harare) 110, 111
Disney corporation 33
Dlamini, Joy 128, 129
Dodge, Martin 239
Doll's House, A (Ibsen) 236, 245
Drama in AIDS Education (DramAidE) 207
DramAidE (Drama in AIDS Education) 127, 207, 208, 212, 213
Drumbeat Communication Initiative Network 36

Du Sautoy, Peter 120
Durban 62, 82, 85, 100, 101, 102, 103, 207, 220, 221
Durden, Emma 132

Eastern Cape (South Africa) 220
Edmiston, Brian, & Jeffrey Wilhelm 148, 159
Edwards, Betty 147, 159
Elam, Keir 254
Ellsworth, Elizabeth 178, 183
Emunah, René, & David Read Johnson 274
Epic Theatre (Brecht) 32
Epskamp, Kees 163
Escobar, Arturo 204
Ethekwini 221
Eyoh, Hansel Ndumbe 55, 56

Fenwick, Tara 63, 64, 65, 66
Fine, Michelle 244, 245
Food and Agricultural Organisation 205, 206
Fortier, Mark 148, 159
Foucault, Michel 240, 241, 249
Fox, Jonathan 145, 149, 159
Frank, Marion 5, 6
Freire, Paulo 47, 67, 84, 88, 114, 150, 159, 241, 254, 260, 277, 278; *Pedagogy of the Oppressed* 47, 67, 150, 159, 254, 278

Gallagher, Kathleen 181
Games for Actors and Non-Actors (Boal) 255, 275
Gauteng (SA province) 220, 253
Gaventa, John, & Andrea Cornwall 111
George, David 211
Ghana xiii, xvi, 187–202
Ghetto Artists (Francistown, Botswana) 35, 36
Giroux, Henry 205, 270, 271, 278
Gladwell, Malcolm xvi, 145, 146, 147, 151, 155, 158, 159
Goran, Hyden 114
Gräbner, Cornelia 130
Grady, Sharon 179, 181, 183
Grahamstown 182
Gramsci, Antonio 273
Green, Paul 239

Haseman, Brad, & John O'Toole 256
HSRC (Human Sciences Research Council) 180, 184, 213
Human Sciences Research Council 180, 213, 223

Ibsen, Henrik, *A Doll's House* 236, 245
Ingwavuma Orphan Care 221, 230
Integrated Regional Development Program (IRDP) 212
InterAction Leadership Programme 49
International Institute for Sustainable Development 48, 54
Irwin, Eleanor 272

Jackson, Adrian 257
Jackson, Michael 149, 159
Jansen, Jonathan D. xvi, 178, 179, 184
Jennings, Sue, Ann Cattanach, Steve Mitchell, Anna Chesner & Brenda Meldrum 255, 261, 262, 263, 264
Johannesburg 36, 150, 159, 251–66, 269–78
Johns Hopkins University 36, 37, 212
Johnson, David Read 274
Johnstone, Keith 151, 159

Kafka, Franz 161
Kamlongera, Christopher 206
Kampala 4, 5, 21, 29
Kentridge, William, *Ubu and the Truth Commission* 237
Kenya xiii
Kerr, David 31, 32, 56, 254; & Stephen Chifunyise 32
Kershaw, Baz 162, 171, 172
Khayalitsha 240, 246
Khoshnood, Kaveh 87, 88
Khoza, Brian 132
Kidd, Ross 254
Kintu, Martin 15, 18, 19, 20
Kistner, Ulrike 179, 180
Kolb, David A. 63, 64, 65, 116
Krog, Antjie 53
Kumba Workshop 55
KwaZulu–Natal 103, 220, 221, 229, 230
Kyakuwa, Julius (Ugandan informant) 7, 18

Lachman, Jamie 169, 220
Landy, Robert 258
Legislative Theatre (Boal) 84
Lesotho xiii, xvi, 145–72, 212, 220, 221, 229, 230
Limpopo 221
Lo, Jacqueline, & Helen Gilbert 84, 90, 93, 94, 104, 106
Ludema, James D. et al. 49
Lutheran Development Service 221, 230, 231

Mabuza, Stanley 94, 95
Macbeth, Douglas 238
Madame and Eve (SA cartoon strip) 275
Madlala, Ntokozo 132
Magalasi, Mufananji 31
Maguire, Patricia 111
Makerere University 4, 17, 27
Makgabaneng (Botswana radio campaign) 37, 38, 39
Malawi xiii, xvi, 31, 32, 33, 34, 40, 41, 43, 187–202, 206
Mamba, Nicholas 92
Mangeni, Patrick 4, 5, 6, 19
Maritz, Johan 166
Marsick, Victoria J. 62
Mbabane (Swaziland) 94, 95
Mbabane Theatre Club 94
Mbaku, John Mukim 113
Mbowa, Rose 5, 6
McCombs, Barbara L., & James E. Pope 121
McLaren, Peter 205
McNiff, Jean, & Jack Whitehead 111, 112
Mda, Zakes 56, 150, 158, 159
Mdlala, Nkululeko 131
Meadows, Grace 265
Mezirow, Jack 63, 64, 65, 66
Michelson, Elana 63, 64
Miles, Matthew B., & A. Michael Huberman 67
Minh-ha, Trinh T. 244
Mityana (Uganda) 29
Monkeybiz Factory Shop 240
Monkeybiz wellness clinic 236, 248
Mooki, Maungo 37, 38
Morris, Gay 64
Motsa, Zodwa 98
Moustakas, Clark 235
Moyo, Arifani 132
Mozambique xiii, 212
Mulago 19, 21
Mwanje, Justus 115
Mwine, Ntare 87, 88
Myerhoff, Barbara, & Jay Ruby 237, 239

Nachmanovitch, Stephen 156, 159
Namibia xiii
National Arts Council 221, 236
National University of Lesotho 150
Ndebele 207
Neelands, Jonothan 116, 177, 183
Nelson, Nici, & Susan Wright 205, 208
Ngema, Mbongeni, *Asinamali* 34
Ng'ombe, James L. 208
Nicholson, Helen 182, 183, 213, 214, 241, 242
Njabulo HIV/AIDS Residency Programme 220, 221, 223, 227
nKwalini and amphitheatre 94, 95, 97, 99, 105, 106
Norwegian Students Academy International Helpfund (SAIH) 212
Ntsangase, Nqobile 132
Nye, Francis Ivan 253

O'Connor, Peter J. 277
O'Neill, Cecily 213, 255, 257, 260, 265, 266
O'Sullivan, Carmel 149, 159
O'Toole, John 209, 210, 256, 257, 261, 265
Obama, Barack 154, 159
Okagbu, Osita 84
Olive Leaf Foundation 269, 270
Oliver, Michael 113
Orleans, Myron 148, 159
Oron, Baron (Ugandan informant) 4, 8, 10, 12, 14, 16, 17, 20, 23, 25
Otukile, Vuyisele 35

Palmer, Gamal 87, 92, 95, 100
Pappas–DeLuca, Katina 38
Parker, Warren 62
Pavis, Patrice 83
Pedagogy of the Oppressed (Freire) 47, 67, 150, 159, 254, 278
Penn, Claire 162
People's Educational Theatre 85, 91
PET artists collective (South Africa) 91, 92, 94, 95, 97, 98, 103, 104, 106
PETA (Filipino theatre group) 32
Pickles, John 249
Pietermaritzburg 127, 129, 142
Plan International (Uganda) 5, 29
Platform Poets 131
PLWHA (People Living with HIV/AIDS) 187, 188, 191, 192, 193, 194, 197, 200, 201, 202
Poltrona, Tortell "Jauma" 220
Prentki, Tim 209, 269, 270, 278
Preston, Sheila 209, 210
Pretoria xvi, 70, 81, 161, 162, 166, 167
Preventing Mother to Child Transmission Project (USAID) 212
Prinsloo, Reineth 166
Project Njabulo 219–32

Rahman, M. Anisur 113, 119
Rahnema, Majid 208, 209, 210
Rainbow of Desire, The (Boal) 251, 255, 257
Rakai District (Uganda) 29
Rasmussen, Björn, & Anna Lena–Ostern 211, 212
Reason, Peter, & Hilary Bradbury 111, 112
Rees, Fran 151, 159
Regional Psychosocial Support Initiative 223, 224, 225
REPSSI (Regional Psychosocial Support Initiative) 224

Richter, Linda, Geoff Foster & Lorraine Sherr 223, 224, 226
Roach, Joseph 99
Rob Smetherham Bereavement Service for Children 220
Rodd, Michael 251

Saaka, Iddi 187
Samba, Emelda Ngufor 48, 58
Sands, Sarah 147
Sartre, Jean-Paul 274
Sayed, Ahmed S. 8, 9
Schechner, Richard 83, 213
Schön, Donald 238
School Health Education Project (Uganda) 4
Schützenberger, Anne Ancelin 277
Shor, Ira 272, 273
Sicherman, Carol 5, 6
Sinyanmanthula (Swaziland) 219
Siwela Sonke dance theatre (Durban) 83, 85, 100, 102
Sophiatown (SA) 252
Soul City Institute (Johannesburg) 36, 37, 38, 39, 40
South Africa xiii, 61–80, 83–108, 127–43, 161–72, 177–84, 207, 219–32, 235–49, 251–66, 269–78
South African Tuberculosis Vaccine Initiative 91
Southern African Development Community (SADC) 212
Soweto 252
Spolin, Viola 151, 159
Steier, Frederick 246
Swaziland xiii, 83–108, 212, 219–32
Swaziland Action Group Against Abuse (SWAGAA) 91
Sweden 220, 221

Tanzania xiii
Taylor, Philip 148, 159, 257, 258, 259, 262
Taylor, Victor E., & Charles Winquist 240
Theatre of the Oppressed (Boal) 53, 54, 55, 149, 150, 158, 254, 260, 272
Theatre Partners (Uganda) 20
Themba Interactive (Johannesburg) xvii, 251–66
Thomas-Slayter, Barbara 117
Thompson, James 165, 169, 214
Trevor Huddleston Memorial Centre 252

Ubu and the Truth Commission (Kentridge) 237
Uchino, Tadashi 211
Uganda xiii, xv, 3–30
UNESCO 203, 205
UNICEF 4, 6, 106, 230
United Nations Decade for Cultural Development 203
United States Agency for International Development (USAID) 212
University of California 187, 188
University of KwaZulu-Natal xvi, 127, 129
University of Malawi 31, 188
University of Pretoria 167, 171
University of Zimbabwe 109

Van den Berg, S. 167
van der Riet, Mary, Angela Hough & Bev Killian 118
van der Stichele, Philippe 206
Vygotsky, Lev Semenovich 276

Walker, Liz, Graeme Reid & Morna Cornell 180
Wheatley, Brandon 94
Wine, Bobi 18
Winter/Summer Institute in Theatre for Development
—See: WSI
Wittgenstein, Ludwig 241
World AIDS Day 2009 236
World Health Organisation 33
World Social Forum (Nairobi) 86
Woza Moya Project 220, 230
WSI (Winter/Summer Institute in Theatre for Development ix, 145, 146, 147, 148, 149, 150, 151, 152, 153, 154, 155, 156, 157, 158

Xhosa 238, 240, 245

Yale School of Drama 86
Yale University 83, 85, 86, 87, 88, 89, 90, 92, 93, 94, 96, 97, 98, 99, 100, 101, 102, 103, 104, 105, 106, 107, 221
Yaounde (Cameroon) 58
Yin, Robert K. 235
YOHO (Youth Health Organisation) 36
Youth Health Organisation (Botswana) 36

Zambia xiii, 31, 32
Zandspruit (SA) xvii, 269–78
Zikalala, Musawenkosi 94, 95, 96, 97, 105
Zimbabwe xiii, 109–22, 207, 212
Zomba (Malawi) 31, 34, 196

Notes for Contributors

Editorial Board

GORDON COLLIER, Im Wiesgarten 9, 35463 Fernwald, GERMANY
Email: Gordon.R.Collier@anglistik.uni-giessen.de

GEOFFREY V. DAVIS, Johanniterstraße 13, 52064 Aachen, GERMANY
Email: davis@anglistik.rwth-aachen.de

CHRISTINE MATZKE, Englische Literaturwissenschaft, Nürnbergerstr. 38, Haus 4, Universität Bayreuth, 95440 Bayreuth, GERMANY
Email: christine.matzke@uni-bayreuth.de

ADEREMI RAJI–OYELADE [pen-name REMI RAJI], Department of English, Faculty of Arts, University of Ìbàdàn, Ìbàdàn 200284, NIGERIA
Email: remraj1@yahoo.com

FRANK SCHULZE–ENGLER, de Ridder Weg 2, 65929 Frankfurt, GERMANY
Email: schulze-engler@nelk.uni-frankfurt.de

WANJIKU WA NGUGI, Helsinki, FINLAND
Email: wanjiku.ngugi@haff.fi

1. SUBMISSIONS. All prospective contributions (articles, creative writing, reports, reviews) and proposals for edited critical collections, as digital files, should be sent as EMAIL ATTACHMENTS to **ALL** of the above-named members of the Editorial Board. Preference is for Word for Windows; **IMPORTANT** – **remove all automatic formatting**).

2. BASIC GUIDELINES FOR INITIAL SUBMISSIONS. Use underlining, NOT *italics*. Include a list of Works Cited. With essays in periodicals and books, include full page-span; with periodicals, include volume and issue number; with translations, include name of translator, the title in the original language, and the date of publication of the original. Use any previous *Matatu* issue as a model for Works Cited, following all of the in-house conventions indicated there. Do NOT use in-text short references. All texts cited or quoted from must

be **footnoted** – include all relevant data (full first and last name of author or editor, title and subtitle, place of publication and publisher; date of first publication and date of edition used).

3. PLEASE NOTE: If the above instructions for basic presentation in 1 and 2 are not followed in essays submitted, the Technical Editor reserves the right either (a) to reject submissions upon receipt or (b) to refuse to accept submissions for consideration until they conform.

4. ABSTRACT AND BIOSKETCH. An abstract of the essay (70–200 words) must be included, along with a brief biosketch for inclusion in the Notes on Contributors (see examples above).

5. STYLESHEET. Should manuscripts, after being accepted for publication, need to be re-submitted on grounds of presentation or layout, the Editors will send contributors a detailed stylesheet.

6. BOOK REVIEWS. Publishers should email Geoffrey V. Davis (see above) attaching details of books that they would like to have reviewed; names and full mailing addresses of appropriate reviewers will then be sent, so that the books can be forwarded.

7. CREATIVE WRITING. Poetry, fiction, and playscripts will, as in the past, be sought out by the Editors of *Matatu* and the Advisory Board, but African writers are, of course, encouraged to submit material for consideration on their own account.

8. THEMES AND TOPICS. Essays on all aspects of African and Afro-Caribbean literature and culture are welcome, as well as reports and interviews on topics of pressing and current concern (many of which can find a place in the occasional "Marketplace" section of *Matatu*).

rodopi

Orders@rodopi.nl—www.rodopi.nl

After "Rwanda"

In Search of a New Ethics

Jean-Paul Martinon

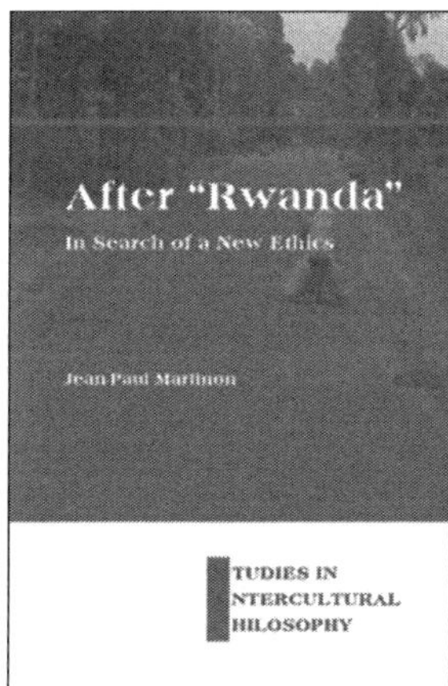

Is writing about peace after the Rwandan Genocide self-defeating? Whether it is the intensity of the massacres, the popularity of the genocide, or the imaginary forms of cruelty, however one looks at it, everything in the Rwandan Genocide appears to defy *once again* the possibility of thinking peace anew. In order to address this problem, this book investigates the work of specific French and Rwandese philosophers in order to renew our understanding of peace today. Through this path-breaking investigation, peace no longer stands for an ideal in the future, but becomes a structure of inter-subjectivity that guarantees that the violence of language always prevails over any other form of violence. This book is the very first monograph in philosophy related to the events of 1994 in Rwanda.

Jean-Paul Martinon is Programme Leader of the MPhil-PhD Programme in Visual Cultures at Goldsmiths College, University of London. He has written monographs on a Victorian workhouse (*Swelling Grounds*, Rear Window, 1995), the idea of the future in the work of Derrida, Malabou and Nancy (*On Futurity*, Palgrave, 2007), the temporal dimension of masculinity (*The End of Man*, Punctum, 2013), and the event of knowledge in museums (*The Curatorial: A Philosophy of Curating*, Bloomsbury, 2013). In each case, he writes in an attempt to make sense of time: its staging in museums, its advent, its gender, its neglect, the ethics that derive from it, and the way it is used and abused to structure human life. www.jeanpaulmartinon.net.

Amsterdam/New York, NY
2013. 308 pp.
(Studies in Intercultural Philosophy 24)
Paper €65,-/US$88,-
E-Book €59,-/US$80,-
ISBN: 978-90-420-3711-3
ISBN: 978-94-012-0967-0

USA/Canada:
Rodopi, 228 East 45th Street, 9E,
New York, NY 10017, USA.
Call Toll-free (US only): T: 1-800-225-3998
F: 1-800-853-3881
All other countries:
Tijnmuiden 7, 1046 AK Amsterdam, The Netherlands
Tel. +31-20-611 48 21 Fax +31-20-447 29 79

Please note that the exchange rate is subject to fluctuations